Upper Gastrointestinal Surgery - Contemporary Techniques and Training

Edited by Rodolfo J. Oviedo

Published in London, United Kingdom

Upper Gastrointestinal Surgery - Contemporary Techniques and Training
http://dx.doi.org/10.5772/intechopen.1006226
Edited by Rodolfo J. Oviedo

Contributors
Aamir Khan, Abhirami Babu, Adel Abou-Mrad, Adel Abou-Mrad, Aman Goyal, Andrés Jonathan Gonzabay De La A, António Albuquerque, Beniamino Pascotto, Beniamino Pascotto, Carlos Luis Malla Vijay, Cinthya Cecilia Ulloa Abad, Evelyn Lucero Capuz Balladares, Javier Aquiles Hidalgo Acosta, Jonathan Gabriel Cobeña Vera, Jorge Eduardo Bejarano Macías, Juan Santiago Azagra, Leonel Amador Zúñiga Arreaga, Leticia del Pilar Barberán Astudillo, Lissette Stephanie Ibarra Velez, Luigi Marano, Mariela Isabel Mora Balladares, Martine Goergen, Miljana Vladimirov, Palak Kirti Jain, Pierre Blanc, Pierre Blanc, Raghav Bansal, Rodolfo J. Oviedo, Rodolfo J. Oviedo, Rosileidy Torres Domínguez, Samridhi Mahajan, Sjaak Pouwels, Vedant Sachin Kasmalkar, Vikas Jain

First published in London, United Kingdom, 2025 by IntechOpen
IntechOpen is the global imprint of INTECHOPEN LIMITED, registered in England and Wales, registration number: 11086078, 167-169 Great Portland Street, London, W1W 5PF, United Kingdom

For EU product safety concerns: IN TECH d.o.o., Prolaz Marije Krucifikse Kozulić 3, 51000 Rijeka, Croatia, info@intechopen.com or visit our website at intechopen.com.

British Library Cataloguing-in-Publication Data
A catalogue record for this book is available from the British Library

Upper Gastrointestinal Surgery - Contemporary Techniques and Training
Edited by Rodolfo J. Oviedo
p. cm.
Print ISBN 978-1-83635-127-6
Online ISBN 978-1-83635-126-9
eBook (PDF) ISBN 978-1-83635-128-3

If disposing of this product, please recycle the paper responsibly.

Meet the editor

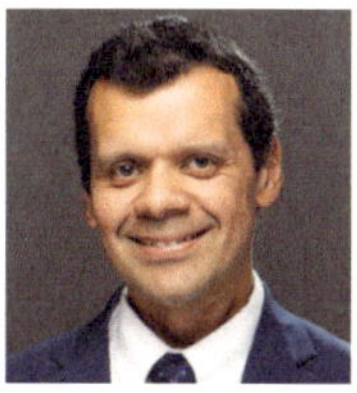

Rodolfo J. Oviedo, MD, FACS, FRCS, FICS, FASMBS, DABS-FPDMBS graduated from medical school at The University of Texas at San Antonio in 2007 and from the Houston Methodist General Surgery Residency Program in 2013. Dr. Oviedo completed an Advanced Minimally Invasive Gastrointestinal and Bariatric Surgery Fellowship at Baptist Hospital of Miami in Miami, Florida, from 2017 to 2018. During this period, he developed his skills as a robotic surgeon. He is a board-certified and fellowship-trained metabolic and bariatric surgeon, as well as a general surgeon. His areas of expertise include robotic metabolic and bariatric surgery, abdominal wall reconstruction, anti-reflux surgery, and interventional bariatric endoscopy. He is a Fellow of the American College of Surgeons (FACS), a Fellow of the Royal College of Surgeons (FRCS), a Fellow of the International College of Surgeons (FICS), and a Fellow of the American Society for Metabolic and Bariatric Surgery (FASMBS). He is a Diplomate of the American Board of Surgery with a Focused Practice Designation in Metabolic and Bariatric Surgery (DABS-FPDMBS). Dr. Oviedo serves on multiple committees at ASMBS, SAGES, ICS, and TROGSS. He has written numerous peer-reviewed manuscripts and book chapters. He is the Deputy Editor of the Journal of Robotic Surgery and an Associate Editor of Obesity Surgery, the official journal of IFSO. Dr. Oviedo is the Medical Director of the Bariatric Surgical Services and Robotics Program at Nacogdoches Medical Center in Nacogdoches, Texas, USA. His commitment to excellence in patient care and the education of the next generation of surgeons continues as a Clinical Professor at the University of Houston's Tilman J. Fertitta Family College of Medicine and Sam Houston State University's College of Osteopathic Medicine. He is honored to serve as CEO of TROGSS - The Robotic Global Surgical Society.

Contents

Preface IX

Section 1
Introduction 1

Chapter 1 3
Introductory Chapter: Technology and Education at the Service of Our Patients
by Rodolfo J. Oviedo

Section 2
Metabolic and Bariatric Surgery 7

Chapter 2 9
Bariatric Acute Abdomen and Its Current Management
by Andrés Jonathan Gonzabay De La A, Javier Aquiles Hidalgo Acosta, Leticia del Pilar Barberán Astudillo, Lissette Stephanie Ibarra Velez, Jorge Eduardo Bejarano Macías, Mariela Isabel Mora Balladares, Cinthya Cecilia Ulloa Abad, Rosileidy Torres Domínguez, Carlos Luis Malla Vijay, Jonathan Gabriel Cobeña Vera, Leonel Amador Zúñiga Arreaga and Evelyn Lucero Capuz Balladares

Chapter 3 25
A Standardized Robotic Roux-en-Y Gastric Bypass
by Pierre Blanc and Adel Abou-Mrad

Chapter 4 33
Robotic One Anastomosis Gastric Bypass
by António Albuquerque

Chapter 5 51
Robotic Roux-en-Y Gastric Bypass: The French Orléans' Way
by Adel Abou-Mrad, Miljana Vladimirov, Aman Goyal, Pierre Blanc, Sjaak Pouwels, Vikas Jain, Beniamino Pascotto, Luigi Marano and Rodolfo J. Oviedo

Section 3
Hepatobiliary and Pancreatic Surgery **63**

Chapter 6 **65**
Choledocholithiasis: Then vs. Now
by Raghav Bansal, Palak Kirti Jain, Abhirami Babu, Vedant Sachin Kasmalkar and Samridhi Mahajan

Chapter 7 **83**
Total Pancreatectomy for Chronic Pancreatitis: Surgical Technique and Recent Advances
by Aamir Khan

Section 4
Upper Gastrointestinal Surgical Oncology **99**

Chapter 8 **101**
Robotic Total and Near-Total (98%) Gastrectomy
by Beniamino Pascotto, Martine Goergen and Juan Santiago Azagra

Preface

The field of upper gastrointestinal (GI) surgery encompasses a vast array of organs, pathologies, and disorders that affect vulnerable patient populations, for which a refined, collaborative, state-of-the-art and evidence-based approach is mandatory. We are no longer allowed to treat patients based on opinion; instead, high-quality literature and evidence take precedence in driving our decisions as specialists who care for those in need and who suffer from upper GI disorders. Inspiring breakthroughs in diagnostic and treatment algorithms for upper GI disorders have proliferated over the last decade, coupled with innovative and visionary techniques currently used to educate our next generation of surgeon leaders who will inherit our mission: to save lives to the best of our ability and with a commitment to excellence and self-improvement. It is in this context that the multidisciplinary and multimodal management of upper GI diseases with surgical and endoscopic approaches takes place while emphasizing the supervised mentorship, education, and graduated skill acquisition for our trainees.

This book comprises a variety of chapters dedicated to presenting state-of-the-art management algorithms and surgical techniques, including robotics, therapeutic endoscopy, and artificial intelligence as adjuncts to human judgment. The book also introduces the concept that surgical education and simulation are of paramount importance in disseminating safe surgical principles in a safe and controlled environment, where repetition, precision, attention to detail, and improvement are emphazised to be effectively applied in surgical practice, yielding optimal outcomes for our patients.

Rodolfo J. Oviedo
University of Houston Tilman J. Fertitta Family College of Medicine,
Houston, Texas, United States

Section 1

Introduction

Chapter 1

Introductory Chapter: Technology and Education at the Service of Our Patients

Rodolfo J. Oviedo

1. Background

The field of upper gastrointestinal (GI) surgery comprises a vast array of organs, pathologies, and disorders that affect vulnerable patient populations and for which a refined, collaborative, state-of-the-art and evidenced-based approach is mandatory [1]. We are no longer allowed to treat patients based on opinion, but on the contrary, high-quality literature and evidence take precedence to drive our decisions as specialists who care for those in need and who suffer from upper GI disorders. Our technological advances over the last few decades should correlate with the quality of education that our trainees in the surgical specialties are receiving based on well-structured curricula at institutions around the globe [2]. Inspiring breakthroughs in diagnostic and treatment algorithms for upper GI disorders have proliferated over the last decade coupled with innovative and visionary techniques currently used to educate our next generation of surgeon leaders who will inherit our mission: to save lives to the best of our ability and with a commitment to excellence and self improvement. It is in this context that the multidisciplinary and multimodal management of upper GI diseases with surgical and endoscopic approaches takes place while emphasizing the supervised mentorship, education, and graduated skill acquisition for our trainees.

2. Surgical education through simulation: A global mission

Surgical education can no longer be justified by the old phrase "See One, Do One, Teach One," especially in the context of the current century and its overwhelming amount of technological advancements such as artificial intelligence, virtual reality, augmented reality, and video-based metric acquisition and evaluation [3]. Simulation-based surgical education plays a vital role in the training of surgical residents, interns, fellows, registrars, and in some cases when resources are available at academic centers, medical students. Several innovative concepts have been developed and recently published based on metric and skills acquisition, competency-based assessment and evaluation, and the interaction between human judgment and experience with computer-based algorithms to train our next generation of specialists in the upper GI tract disorders. Such surgical education curricula are based on updated concepts currently utilized by master educators to provide innovative solutions with limited resources in many cases, and with the human element at the core of what is taught rather than the technology itself.

3. Metabolic and bariatric surgery

The superspecialty of metabolic and bariatric surgery (MBS) has paved the way to introduce several innovations including robotic surgery and endo bariatrics with an integral treatment with anti-obesity medications. Such a comprehensive management approach has been shown to have a protective effect on different types of cancer [4]. MBS experts work in a team with other obesity medicine consultants and allied health professionals to provide patients with an individualized and tailored approach to their treatment including endoscopic, laparoscopic, robotic, primary versus revisional, and medical therapy to achieve optimal results with continuity of care and close follow-up.

4. Upper GI oncology

The most advanced techniques in upper GI oncology have advanced with the robotic approach and the use of adjuncts such as artificial intelligence in real time as well as fluorescence imaging assessment of perfusion and anastomosis creation. At the same time, surgical oncology education and curriculum development to train surgeons on these specialized operations have been developed at many programs around the world and have been implemented at academic institutions and simulation centers.

5. Benign upper GI pathology

Benign upper GI diseases require surgical and endoscopic treatment options with the latest evidence-based concepts and lessons learned by experts in the field. Challenging problems such as choledocholithiasis and gastrointestinal bleeding are currently treated with minimally invasive technologies and approaches including advanced therapeutic endoscopic techniques.

6. Surgical training curricula: Measurable competencies

The most innovative, dynamic, outside-the-box curricula used to train residents, interns, registrars, fellows, surgeons in practice, and in some cases, medical students with attention to skills acquisition and competency mastery are illustrated by the CARS Curriculum (*Competency-Based Assessment of Robotic Surgery Skills*) [5]. This is a key mission for its authors and educators: to inspire our current and future educators to develop training curricula and an objective evaluation system to train the next generation of surgical leaders.

7. Conclusion and acknowledgement

The maintenance of certification and acquisition of skills to master the minimally invasive surgical and endoscopic techniques for upper GI disorders and diseases is essential in our current era and a necessity for our students, trainees, and surgeons in practice. After all, this desire to keep improving every day for the benefit of our patients is at the core of what we do. Special thanks and acknowledgement to the leaders and members of TROGSS - The Robotic Global Surgical Society for their commitment and passion for the global mission of #surgicaleducationforall. To all of them, I offer my deepest gratitude and admiration.

Author details

Rodolfo J. Oviedo[1,2,3,4]

1 Department of Surgery, Nacogdoches Medical Center, Nacogdoches, TX, USA

2 University of Houston Tilman J. Fertitta Family College of Medicine, Houston, TX, USA

3 Sam Houston State University College of Osteopathic Medicine, Conroe, TX, USA

4 TROGSS - The Robotic Global Surgical Society, Orléans, France

*Address all correspondence to: roviedo3@central.uh.edu

References

[1] Pędziwiatr M, Mavrikis J, Witowski J, Adamos A, Major P, Nowakowski M, et al. Current status of enhanced recovery after surgery (ERAS) protocol in gastrointestinal surgery. Medical Oncology. 2018;**35**(6):95. DOI: 10.1007/s12032-018-1153-0

[2] Gleason A, Harrington C, Alvi S, Han SM, Sullivan ME, Aziz H. Evaluating general surgical residency education structure and incorporation of the resident as educator model. Journal of Surgical Education. 2022;**79**(6):1387-1393. DOI: 10.1016/j.jsurg.2022.05.020 Epub 2022 Jun 18

[3] Sinha A, West A, Vasdev N, Sooriakumaran P, Rane A, Dasgupta P, et al. Current practises and the future of robotic surgical training. The Surgeon. 2023;**21**(5):314-322. DOI: 10.1016/j.surge.2023.02.006. Epub 2023 Mar 15

[4] Playdon MC, Hardikar S, Karra P, Hoobler R, Ibele AR, Cook KL, et al. Metabolic and bariatric surgery and obesity pharmacotherapy for cancer prevention: Current status and future possibilities. Journal of the National Cancer Institute. Monographs. 2023;**2023**(61):68-76. DOI: 10.1093/jncimonographs/lgad003

[5] Elzein SM, Corzo MP, Tomey D, et al. Development and initial experience of a novel competency-based assessment of robotic surgery skills (CARS) scale for general surgery residents. Global Surgical Education. 2024;**3**:70. DOI: 10.1007/s44186-024-00265-2

Section 2

Metabolic and Bariatric Surgery

Chapter 2

Bariatric Acute Abdomen and Its Current Management

Andrés Jonathan Gonzabay De La A,
Javier Aquiles Hidalgo Acosta, Leticia del Pilar Barberán Astudillo,
Lissette Stephanie Ibarra Velez, Jorge Eduardo Bejarano Macías,
Mariela Isabel Mora Balladares, Cinthya Cecilia Ulloa Abad,
Rosileidy Torres Domínguez, Carlos Luis Malla Vijay,
Jonathan Gabriel Cobeña Vera, Leonel Amador Zúñiga Arreaga
and Evelyn Lucero Capuz Balladares

Abstract

Bariatric acute abdomen is a serious complication that requires diagnosis in the first few hours for surgical resolution. Its cause is most often due to the formation of internal hernias, ulcers, perforations, and volvulus, which leads to the performance of a revision procedure for its management and resolution. Postoperative complications in bariatric surgery are directly associated with mortality and surgical reintervention; for this reason, it is necessary to recognize all the complications that occur during the trans-surgical or post-surgical period. Bariatric surgery is the most performed surgery in Europe with 50,000 procedures per year. According to these data, it continues to be underused, in many cases due to fear of complications, so France would need 200 years to operate on all patients with obesity. Perioperative mortality ranged from 0.03 to 0.2%. Robotic surgery represents a major advance in the management of bariatric and acute abdominal surgery, allowing complications to be assessed and treated using revision procedures and new minimally invasive repair techniques.

Keywords: abdomen, acute, bariatrics, bariatric surgery, bariatric medicine

1. Introduction

Bariatric acute abdomen is a serious complication that requires diagnosis in the first few hours for surgical resolution. Its cause is most often due to the formation of internal hernias, ulcers, perforations and volvulus, which leads to the performance of a revision procedure for its management and resolution.

Complications of bariatric surgery are exceptional circumstances that may occur intra- and postoperatively; therefore, this chapter is justified due to the role that bariatric surgery plays as the most performed surgical procedure for the management of obesity, type 2 diabetes mellitus and dysmetabolic syndrome, which makes it necessary to recognize the acute and chronic complications of bariatric surgery, including acute abdomen, and the importance of its current treatment [1, 2].

There are acute complications such as bleeding that may occur during surgery or in the immediate postoperative period. In many cases, blood transfusions or medications such as tranexamic acid are necessary to reduce bleeding, until reintervention for revision surgery is performed [3, 4]. Other acute complications are anastomotic leaks that can cause chemical peritonitis or bariatric acute abdomen [5, 6].

Chronic events of bariatric surgery include internal hernias, abdominal wall hernia, cholelithiasis, short bowel syndrome, digestive disorders and malnutrition [7, 8].

Weight gain after bariatric surgery may be greater in some techniques, for example, patients undergoing sleeve gastrectomy (SG) have greater weight gain after surgery compared to other techniques such as Roux-en-Y surgery [9].

Diagnostic imaging studies, such as abdominal computed tomography (CT), abdominal ultrasound and radiographs, are used to visualize free fluid in the abdominal cavity or lesions in abdominal organs. Plain abdominal CT followed by intravenous contrast is the most commonly used imaging in acute abdomen and is positive in 73% of cases. Petersens hernia and other hernias are diagnosed by imaging signs, but in some cases the diagnosis is necessary by laparoscopy or exploratory laparotomy [10].

Abdominal computed tomography is the most accurate test with the presence of imaging findings such as the whirlpool sign, which means rotation of the mesenteric vessels in the axial section with opacity of the mesenteric fat, tapering of the superior mesenteric vein, hooked intestine sign and inversion of the mesenteric arteries and veins [11, 12].

Postoperative complications in bariatric surgery are directly associated with mortality and surgical reintervention; for this reason, it is necessary to recognize all the complications that occur during the trans-surgical or post-surgical period [13].

Bariatric surgery, the most commonly performed surgery in Europe with 50,000 procedures per year, is still underused, often due to fear of complications, and France would need 200 years to operate on all obese patients. Perioperative mortality ranged from 0.03 to 0.2% [14, 15].

Bariatric acute abdomen is a serious complication, the diagnosis of which is based on clinical findings. Timely treatment during the first 24 hours consists of revision surgery. In cases of internal hernias, ulcers, perforations, volvulus and acute abdomen, treatment consists of peritoneal lavage for peritonitis, intestinal resection in cases of necrosis and conversion to other techniques for closing leaks, in addition to the participation of a multidisciplinary team for postoperative management [16].

The objective of this research is to describe bariatric acute abdomen and its current management.

2. Methodology

A literature review was conducted on the topic in Spanish and English, generating two research questions: What is the management of bariatric acute abdomen? and What are the complications of bariatric surgery? Databases, such as PubMed, Mendeley, Google Scholar and Web of Science, were used. Through a random systematic search, 59 articles published in the last 5 years were obtained, which included: clinical trials, systematic reviews, meta-analysis and observational studies on the research topic.

3. Complications of sleeve gastrectomy

Failure of sleeve gastrectomy may present early complications, such as gastrointestinal bleeding, fistulas, gastric perforation, nausea, vomiting and epigastric pain (**Table 1**). Late complications include gastroesophageal reflux, nutritional deficiencies, ulcers, stenosis and chronic gastritis. Sleeve gastrectomy stenosis is a late complication, and its management includes the use of upper gastrointestinal endoscopy, which is essential in balloon dilation, with a success rate of 90% [17].

Gastric leak secondary to sleeve gastrectomy occurs within 6 days after surgery. Gastrocutaneous fistulas may persist chronically and transform into gastropleural fistulas. Endoscopic treatment is performed by stenting, endoscopic clipping, Over-The-Scope or endoscopic suturing [18].

Gastrocutaneous fistula after sleeve gastrectomy occurs in 1–2% and surgical treatment consists of primary repair of the gastric fistula and gastrojejunostomy or conversion to Roux-en-Y gastric bypass (RYGB), while patients treated endoscopically undergo suturing, stenting, dilation and clipping [19].

Digestive endoscopy is useful for the diagnosis and treatment of stricture, leak, choledocholithiasis, gastric sleeve stenosis or eroded anastomosis. During diagnostic laparoscopy, the need for open surgery can be determined in the presence of other complications such as intestinal intussusception [20].

Author	Population	Type of complication	Recommendation management	Level of evidence
Petrucciani et al. [5]	120 pregnant women with a history of bariatric surgery underwent emergency surgery, of which (n: 50 cases) were secondary to complications of bariatric surgery.	Internal hernia was the most frequent complication (n:26), intestinal intussusception (n:10), intestinal obstruction (n:2), adjustable gastric band slippage (n:3), intestinal volvulus (n:3), gastric or jejunal perforation (n:2) and other complications (n:4). Maternal death accounted for 2.5% (n:3) and fetal death for 7.5% (n:9).	Availability of multidisciplinary experts, including bariatric and digestive surgeons. Rapid surgical exploration is mandatory in the presence of clinical and radiological signs of bariatric acute abdomen in pregnancy.	Intermediate
Kermansaravi et al. [6]	Leaks after single anastomosis gastric bypass 410 leaks in 44,318 patients	The most frequently performed procedure was peritoneal lavage and drainage (with or without T-tube placement) in 30.8% of patients, followed by conversion to Roux-en-Y gastric bypass in 9.6% of patients.	62.1% of patients with leaks underwent another surgery.	High

Table 1.
The management of complications included revision surgery with surgical exploration, maternal death is one of the most serious complications that occur due to increased fertility after bariatric surgery and anatomical alterations. It is relevant to consider the history of bariatric surgery in pregnant women with signs of acute abdomen [5, 6].

4. Complications of Roux-en-Y gastric bypass

Roux-en-Y gastric bypass is the most frequently performed bariatric surgery, one of its main complications being marginal ulcers of the duodenojejunal or gastrojejunal anastomosis [21, 22]. Perforated gastrojejunal ulcer is a surgical emergency that can have consequences such as acute peritonitis [23].

Internal hernia is a complication that can be acute and occurs due to the passage of tissue through the defect, which can cause intestinal obstruction, necrosis, perforation and peritonitis [24].

There are three types of internal hernias that occur after bariatric surgery: (1) mesenteric defect hernia, (2) hernia through the transverse mesocolic defect and (3) Petersens hernia, which occur by different mechanisms, such as the lack of space closure, excessive weight loss and increase in the size of the defect, causing strangulation of the intestinal loops and sometimes requiring intestinal resection that can trigger short bowel syndrome [25, 26].

A rare internal hernia is also described, located at the Brolin point, known as small bowel hernia, which is located between this point and the anastomosis [27] and is considered a late complication because it usually occurs after discharge. Petersens

Presentation time after bariatric surgery	Type of repair	Management	Sex, age	Presentation
2 months post Roux-en-Y gastric bypass	Laparoscopic	Reduction of the loop, resection of the gangrenous loop and closure of the defect	44-year-old woman	Abdominal pain of 4-day duration
Petersens hernia after abdominoplasty, 2.5 years after laparoscopic Roux-en-Y gastric bypass	Midline laparotomy	Excision of 30 cm of necrotic jejunum and side-to-side jejunojejunal anastomosis, adhesiolysis, closure of Petersens space with 3/0 Vicryl	42-year-old woman	24 hours of diffuse abdominal pain radiating to the left flank, nausea and vomiting that occurred 3 days after the abdominoplasty
Petersens space hernia repair 5 years after mini gastric bypass	Laparoscopic	Conversion to Roux-en-Y gastric bypass and closure of mesenteric defect with continuous 2/0 silk suture	Man 26 years old	Intermittent and chronic abdominal pain
Petersens hernia in a pregnant woman 8 years after bariatric surgery	Emergency laparoscopy	Bowel resection, closure of the gastric pouch, intestinal anastomosis and Stamm gastrostomy and closure of the space	42-year-old female, 34 weeks pregnant	Colicky abdominal pain in the epigastrium, radiating to the right hypochondrium.

Description. Chronic complications can also cause bariatric acute abdomen between 2 months and 8 years after surgery, and its management includes laparoscopic revision surgery with resection, conversion to another technique, gastrostomy and closure of the Petersens space [37–40].

Table 2.
Clinical characteristics and presentation time of bariatric acute abdomen secondary to Petersens hernia and its surgical management.

hernia and mesenteric defect hernia cause intestinal obstruction, which can occur several years after bariatric surgery [10, 28]. The diagnosis of both pathologies is made by CT and diagnostic laparoscopy. Treatment includes routine laparoscopic closure of mesenteric defects with staples to prevent reopening [29].

The incidence of internal hernia in bariatric surgery is between 0.2 and 9.0% and Petersens hernia has an incidence of 0.1 to 0.02%, both characterized by abdominal pain, intestinal obstruction or acute abdomen, months or years after surgery, increasing the need for new surgery or admission to the intensive care unit, even patients who undergo prophylactic closure of the Petersens space may continue to present Petersens hernia [30–32]. The risk of internal hernia after bariatric surgery tends to increase over time, the cumulative incidence is 4.80% at 3 years (95% CI: 4.59–5.02%) and at the 13th year of follow-up, the cumulative incidence may be up to 12% (95% CI: 11.30–12.70%) [24].

Currently, routine closure of the defect is recommended to avoid this complication [33], with a reduction observed in cases following bariatric surgery; for example, after laparoscopic Roux-en-Y gastric bypass, there is a reduction in the incidence of intestinal obstruction when Petersens space closure is performed [34].

A multicenter randomized controlled trial compared both techniques (closure of all defects versus no closure) with follow-up for 25 months and observed a significant increase in major complications in the closure of all defects group, associated with a higher risk of early small bowel obstruction odds ratio 1.55, 95% CI 1.01–2.39 [35]. Each management should be individualized due to situations such as the size of the defect or the body mass index (BMI) of the patients, since Petersens space herniorrhaphy is not free of complications [36].

There are different treatment options, see **Table 2**, which include the type of repair through open, laparoscopic, endoscopic, robotic or hybrid approaches. For defect closure, closure methods include fascial closure, mesh closure and bonding [41].

5. Complications in biliopancreatic diversion with duodenal switch

This surgery is reserved for patients with BMI > 50 super obese, which consists of a sleeve gastrectomy with laparoscopic duodeno-ileal anastomosis, the procedure consists of a duodeno-ileal bypass and jejuno-ileal anastomosis, with sleeve gastrectomy when weight loss or decompensated diabetes does not show remission after other surgeries (**Table 3**) [45].

Biliopancreatic diversion with duodenal switch has acute and chronic complications, such as: diarrhea, nausea or vomiting, osteoporosis and biliary lithiasis, the latter being a common cause of cholecystectomy, in addition, dumping syndrome, malnutrition, vitamin deficiency, intestinal obstruction, gastric perforation, internal hernias, hypoglycemia and perforated ulcer [46].

6. Complications of laparoscopic gastric bypass with single banded anastomosis

Laparoscopic gastric bypass with single banded anastomosis is a technique that adds banding to the gastric pouch. In a retrospective study of 86 patients undergoing this procedure between 2018 and 2020, operative outcomes showed an average operative time of 48 minutes with 3.4% early complications and 2.3% late complications.

Authors	Intervention	Number of patients (n)	Results	Level of evidence
Zhang et al. [42]	Robotic bariatric surgery compared to laparoscopic bariatric surgery for obesity	7239 cases of robotic surgery and 203,181 cases of laparoscopic surgery	Longer operative time [P < 0.01] and lower mortality for robotic surgery [OR 2.40; 95% CI (1.24–4.64); P = 0.009]	Systematic review and meta-analysis
Bertoni et al. [43]	Robot-assisted versus laparoscopic revisional bariatric surgery	29,890 patients (2459 in the robotic group)	No significant differences in perioperative complications, hospital stay or operating time	Systematic review and meta-analysis
Nasser et al. [44]	Comparative analysis of bariatric surgery [sleeve gastrectomy (SG) and Roux-en-Y gastric bypass (RYGB)] performed by robotic versus laparoscopic revision and their perioperative outcomes	17,012 patients underwent revisional gastric sleeve with 15,935 (93.7%) laparoscopic and 1077 (6.3%) robotic, and 12,442 patients underwent revisional Roux-en-Y bypass with 11,212 (90.1%) laparoscopic and 1230 (9.9%) robotic.	The robotic approach was associated with a longer operating time (P < 0.01). The length of hospital stay was longer in the robotic group for OS (P < 0.01). Morbidity was higher in robotic SG compared with laparoscopic SG 6.7% vs. 4.5% (P < 0.01). Robotic RYGB was associated with comparable overall morbidity to laparoscopic RYGB (9.3% versus 11.6% P = 0.07).	Comparative study

Description: The use of robotic surgery in the context of bariatric acute abdomen presents good results, and it can be used in revision surgeries. The comparison showed that laparoscopic surgery has a larger population of patients studied due to the wide implementation of the technique, becoming the most used procedure, morbidity depends on the type of surgery performed, with lower morbidity in laparoscopic sleeve gastrectomy revision and RYGB by robotic surgery, in addition to a longer operating time and lower mortality, making the robotic approach a useful tool for the management of bariatric acute abdomen.

Table 3.
Comparison of morbidity, mortality and complications of bariatric surgery according to the laparoscopic or robotic approach [42–44].

One patient required reoperation due to acute abdomen on account of intra-abdominal hemorrhage.

Laparoscopic gastric bypass with single anastomosis can be performed with or without wrapping, both techniques are recognized as simple and safe, with biliary reflux being the most frequent complication, which is resolved by Nissen fundoplication with the remaining stomach as an antireflux valve [47, 48].

7. Early complications of bariatric surgery

In the intraoperative and immediate postoperative periods, the most frequent complications are intestinal perforation, hemorrhages and suture dehiscence, and are characterized by shock, sudden hypotension, tachycardia and hypoperfusion. In the immediate postoperative period, complications may manifest with abdominal pain that does not improve with intravenous analgesics, dyspnea, hypoxemia, hemodynamic instability, metabolic alterations, hyperglycemia, hypoglycemia, metabolic acidosis and acute anemia.

Treatment of acute complications in this type of surgery should be performed immediately according to the patient's clinical condition and the results of additional tests. In cases of shock associated with hypovolemia, transfusion of blood products is recommended if the hemoglobin value is less than 7 mg/dL or if there is active bleeding with hemodynamic instability. Platelet transfusion is indicated in the presence of thrombocytopenia plus active bleeding, fresh frozen plasma or cryoprecipitates if coagulation times or fibrinogen is altered, requiring management in the intensive care unit, gastroenterology and nutritional support.

During the perioperative period, early complications occur, such as upper or lower gastrointestinal bleeding, sepsis, malnutrition, overfeeding, fluid and electrolyte imbalance, metabolic disorders, ileus, intestinal obstruction, among others, so identifying early complications that occur after bariatric surgery is essential and its diagnosis will be based on laboratory tests with metabolic or electrolyte alterations. Other complementary studies include upper and lower gastrointestinal endoscopy, simple and contrast-enhanced abdominal tomography and abdominal ultrasound, all of which contribute to diagnostic accuracy. In the first 30 postoperative days, acute internal hernias may occur with an incidence between 0.4 and 1.2% [49].

8. Late complications of bariatric surgery

Late complications occur after discharge, including internal hernias such as Petersens hernia and mesenteric defect hernia, which may cause intestinal obstruction and present late until years after bariatric surgery [10, 28]. Diagnosis of both pathologies is made by CT or diagnostic laparoscopy. Treatment includes routine laparoscopic closure of mesenteric defects with staples to prevent reopening [29].

Acute bariatric abdomen is a serious complication that can also be delayed due to the anatomical alterations after surgery, so timely diagnosis and treatment during the first hours is necessary, with surgical resolution, in internal hernias, ulcers, perforations, and volvulus, being the most frequently reported complications. A large percentage of patients require a new procedure with peritoneal lavage for peritonitis or conversion to other techniques for the management of leaks, in addition to a multidisciplinary team for their management (**Figures 1** and **2**).

In cases of hemodynamic instability with perforation and hemorrhage, open reintervention surgical treatment should be considered, since these patients develop hypovolemic shock [4].

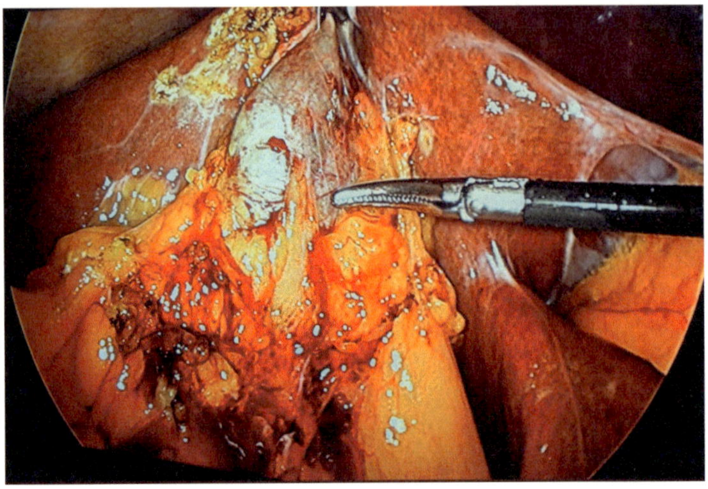

Figure 1.
Intraoperative image of successful laparoscopic cholecystectomy in a patient with a history of bariatric surgery who presented cholelithiasis.

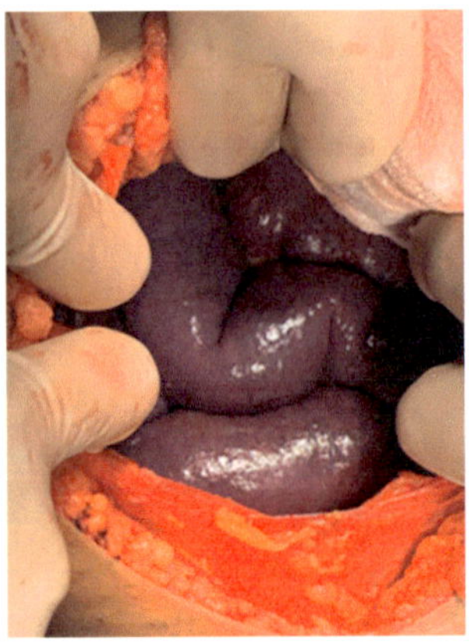

Figure 2.
Intraoperative exploratory laparotomy image in a patient with acute abdomen, mesenteric ischemia is observed.

The routine use of the nutritional guideline in critically obese patients should be managed strictly and dynamically by parenteral and oral routes at the corresponding times, according to their evolution [49].

Current management of Petersens hernia, clinical manifestations, presentation time after bariatric surgery and type of repair, the possibility of presenting an internal hernia after bariatric surgery is greater if the defect is not closed, and there may be intestinal necrosis with the need for resection, ostomies and closure of the Petersens defect. Surgical treatment is performed by open or laparoscopic surgery [37–40].

9. Abdominal wall hernia and bariatric surgery

Management of abdominal wall hernia is performed according to the surgical situation, in three stages: (1) repair before bariatric surgery, (2) repair after surgery and (3) simultaneous repair and will depend on each case according to the size of the hernia. Concomitant treatment is associated with lower probabilities of surgical site infection, reintervention and seromas. Complications in abdominal wall hernia consist of hematomas, seromas and surgical site infections [50].

Ventral hernias can be repaired with simple suture, synthetic mesh (polypropylene) and biological mesh depending on the defect. The recurrence rate is about 25.7% in the suture group, 14.3% in the biological mesh group and 1.1% in the synthetic mesh group. Hernias at the trocar insertion site are a rare complication in bariatric surgery, but it is important to mention it [51, 52].

Robotic repair techniques for abdominal wall hernia consist of the creation of myocutaneous flaps that are composed of skin, subcutaneous tissue, fascia and muscle. They are used to cover large defects in the skin, through complex robotic reconstruction techniques of the abdominal wall, with the placement of fixed mesh on the abdominal wall. First primary closure of peritoneal defects is performed, then the mesh is superimposed for defects of 4 to 5 cm. Adhesiolysis and reduction of the hernial sac may be necessary. Extraperitoneal repair of the defect avoids complications, such as intestinal adhesions, erosion of the mesh and enterocutaneous fistulas secondary to direct contact between the mesh and the intestine, hernioplasty is performed using a totally extraperitoneal technique [53].

10. Conclusions

In the presence of signs of peritoneal irritation or persistent abdominal pain, recognizing the immediate, early and late complications that can cause bariatric acute abdomen is of vital importance, due to the need for multidisciplinary management to resolve surgical emergencies, including acute hemorrhage, anastomotic leak, intestinal obstruction, intestinal necrosis and intra-abdominal infections, which are the main causes of bariatric acute abdomen.

The management of bariatric acute abdomen requires a surgical approach, as well as medical treatment with resuscitation, hemodynamic support, antibiotics, nutrition and recovery in intensive care unit, giving priority to the control of hemorrhage, infection and the resolution of surgical complications with laparoscopic, robotic or open revision exploration.

Robotic surgery represents a major advance in the management of bariatric surgery and acute abdomen, allowing complications to be evaluated and treated through revision procedures and new minimally invasive repair techniques.

Acknowledgements

I thank my mother for her unconditional support during my years of study.

CRediT author statement

Hidalgo Javier: Conceptualization and resources, Gonzabay Andrés: Methodology, Barberán Leticia: Software and formal analysis, Ibarra Lissette: Data curation, Bejarano Jorge: Writing original draft, Hidalgo Javier: Revision and editing of the original draft, Mora Mariela: Visualization, Ulloa Cinthya: Research, Torres Rosileidy:

Supervision, Malla Carlos: Project management, Zúñiga Leonel: Writing the final draft, Cobeña Jonathan: Revision of the final manuscript, Capuz Evelin: Final acceptance of the chapter, Gonzabay Andres: Acquisition of funds and translation.

Conflict of interest

The authors declare no conflict of interest.

Acronyms and abbreviations

CT	computed tomography
SG	sleeve gastrectomy
RYGB	Roux-en-Y gastric bypass

DOI: http://dx.doi.org/10.5772/intechopen.1009469

Author details

Andrés Jonathan Gonzabay De La A[1], Javier Aquiles Hidalgo Acosta[2]*, Leticia del Pilar Barberán Astudillo[1], Lissette Stephanie Ibarra Velez[3], Jorge Eduardo Bejarano Macías[4], Mariela Isabel Mora Balladares[5], Cinthya Cecilia Ulloa Abad[6], Rosileidy Torres Domínguez[7], Carlos Luis Malla Vijay[2], Jonathan Gabriel Cobeña Vera[8], Leonel Amador Zúñiga Arreaga[9] and Evelyn Lucero Capuz Balladares[10]

1 General Hospital of the North of Guayaquil, Ecuador

2 University of Guayaquil, Ecuador

3 Omni Hospital, Guayaquil, Ecuador

4 University Catholic of Santiago de Guayaquil, Ecuador

5 Urban Health Center, Daule, Ecuador

6 Municipal Social Action of the Cuenca, Ecuador

7 Matilde Hidalgo of Procel Hospital, Guayaquil, Ecuador

8 Emergency Medical Service, Health Center Type C, La Concordia, Ecuador

9 Higher Institute Bolivariano Technology, Guayaquil, Ecuador

10 Regional Autonomous University of the Andes UNIANDES, Quito, Ecuador

*Address all correspondence to: jahidalgoacosta@hotmail.com

References

[1] Larsen M, Kozarek R. Therapeutic endoscopy for the treatment of post-bariatric surgery complications. World Journal of Gastroenterology. 2022;**28**(2):199-215. DOI: 10.3748/wjg.v28.i2.199

[2] Hu L, Ma L, Xia X, Ying T, Zhou M, Zou S, et al. Efficacy of bariatric surgery in the treatment of women with obesity and polycystic ovary syndrome. The Journal of Clinical Endocrinology and Metabolism. 2022;**107**(8):e3217-e3229. DOI: 10.1210/clinem/dgac294

[3] JWH t'H, Noordman BJ, JMA W, Biter LU, SJC V, Birnie E, et al. Peroperative administration of tranexamic acid in sleeve gastrectomy to reduce hemorrhage: A double-blind randomized controlled trial. Surgical Endoscopy. 2023;**37**(10):7455-7463. DOI: 10.1007/s00464-023-10232-5

[4] Hossain N, Kaur V, Mahran M, Quddus A, Mukhopadhyay S, Shah A, et al. Intra-operative tranexamic acid administration significantly decreases incidence of postoperative bleeding without increasing venous thromboembolism risk after laparoscopic sleeve gastrectomy: A retrospective cohort study of over 400 patients. Obesity Surgery. 2024;**34**(2):396-401. DOI: 10.1007/s11695-023-07021-3

[5] Petrucciani N, Martini F, Kassir R, Juglard G, Hamid C, Boudrie H, et al. Internal hernia after one anastomosis gastric bypass (OAGB): Lessons learned from a retrospective series of 3368 consecutive patients undergoing OAGB with a biliopancreatic limb of 150 cm. Obesity Surgery. 2021;**31**(6):2537-2544. DOI: 10.1007/s11695-021-05269-1

[6] Kermansaravi M, Kassir R, Valizadeh R, Parmar C, Davarpanah Jazi AH, Shahmiri SS, et al. Management of leaks after gastric bypass with one anastomosis: An updated systematic review and meta-analysis of 44,318 patients. International Journal of Surgery. 2023;**109**(5):1497-1508. DOI: 10.1097/JS9.0000000000000346

[7] Araki S, Shani Levi C, Abutbul Vered S, Solt I, Rozen GS. Pregnancy after bariatric surgery: Effects of personalized nutrition counseling on pregnancy outcomes. Clinical Nutrition. 2022;**41**(2):288-297. DOI: 10.1016/j.clnu.2021.11.035

[8] Abualsel A et al. Internal hernia post-single anastomosis gastric bypass: Case series with review of literature. The Surgery Journal. 2024;**10**:e31-e35

[9] Akpinar EO, Liem RSL, Nienhuijs SW, Greve JWM, Marang-van de Mheen PJ. Dutch audit for treatment of obesity research group. Weight recurrence after sleeve gastrectomy versus Roux-en-Y gastric bypass: A propensity score matched nationwide analysis. Surgical Endoscopy. 2023;**37**(6):4351-4359. DOI: 10.1007/s00464-022-09785-8

[10] Blockhuys M, Gypen B, Heyman S, Valk J, van Sprundel F, Hendrickx L. Internal hernia after laparoscopic gastric bypass: Effect of closure of the Petersen defect - single-center study. Obesity Surgery. 2019;**29**(1):70-75. DOI: 10.1007/s11695-018-3472-9

[11] Permekerlis A, Gemousakaki E, Tepelidis C, Fotiadis P. Internal herniation causing double obstruction of the small bowel and urinary tract: A rare case presentation. Cureus. 2024;**16**(7):e65483. DOI: 10.7759/cureus.65483

[12] Pedro L-M, González-Valverde Francisco M, Antonio A-M-B. Petersen's space hernia in a patient who underwent gastric bypass. Circle [online magazine]. 2020;**88**(6):772-775. Available from: http://www.scielo.org.mx/scielo.php?script=sci_arttext&pid=S2444-054X2020000600772&lng=es. Epub 08-Nov-2021. DOI: 10.24875/ciru.20000905

[13] Bordonaro V, Brizi MG, Lanza F, et al. Role of CT scan in differentiating internal hernia from specific abdominal pain after Roux-en-Y gastric bypass: The experience of a single, high-volume center. Updates in Surgery. 2020;**72**:1115-1124. DOI: 10.1007/s13304-020-00767-w

[14] Palermo M, Nedelcu M. Complications in bariatric surgery. Journal of Laparoendoscopic & Advanced Surgical Techniques. 2021;**A31**:139-140. DOI: 10.1089/lap.2020.0910

[15] Arterburn DE, Telem DA, Kushner RF, Courcoulas AP. Benefits and risks of bariatric surgery in adults: A review. JAMA. 2020;**324**(9):879-887. DOI: 10.1001/jama.2020.12567

[16] De Simone B, Chouillard E, Ramos AC, Donatelli G, Pintar T, Gupta R, et al. Operative management of acute abdomen after bariatric surgery in the emergency setting: The OBA guidelines. World Journal of Emergency Surgery : WJES. 2022;**17**(1):51. DOI: 10.1186/s13017-022-00452-w. Erratum in: World J Emerg Surg. 2022 Nov 7;17(1):58. DOI: 10.1186/s13017-022-00460-w

[17] Masood M, Low DE, Deal SB, Kozarek RA. Endoscopic management of post-sleeve gastrectomy complications. Journal of Clinical Medicine. 2024;**13**(7):2011. DOI: 10.3390/jcm13072011

[18] Negm S, Mousa B, Shafiq A, Abozaid M, Allah EA, Attia A, et al. Endoscopic management of refractory leak and gastro-cutaneous fistula after laparoscopic sleeve gastrectomy: A randomized controlled trial. Surgical Endoscopy. 2023;**37**(3):2173-2181. DOI: 10.1007/s00464-022-09748-z

[19] Parkash O, Sohail Z, Khalid N. Endoscopic stent placement for the management of gastro-pleural and gastro-cutaneous fistula post laparoscopic sleeve gastrectomy: A case report. Journal of Medical Case Reports. 2023;**17**(1):461. DOI: 10.1186/s13256-023-04200-9

[20] Jamshidi M, Rahimi B, Gilani N. Laparoscopic and open surgery methods in managing surgical intussusceptions: A randomized clinical trial of postoperative complications. Asian Journal of Endoscopic Surgery. 2022;**15**(1):56-62. DOI: 10.1111/ases.12965

[21] Chang SH, Popov VB, Thompson CC. Endoscopic balloon dilation for treatment of sleeve gastrectomy stenosis: A systematic review and meta-analysis. Gastrointestinal Endoscopy. 2020;**91**(5):989-1002.e4. DOI: 10.1016/j.gie.2019.11.034

[22] Ferrer-Márquez M, García-Redondo M, Maturana-Ibáñez V, Estébanez-Ferrero B, Fernández-Alonso A, Rubio-Gil F, et al. Bile reflux and marginal ulcers after one-anastomosis gastric bypass (OAGB). A narrative review. Cirugía Española (Engl Ed). 2023;**101**(Suppl 4):S69-S75. DOI: 10.1016/j.cireng.2023.04.006

[23] Fry BT, Finks JF. Abdominal pain after roux-en-Y gastric bypass: A review. JAMA Surgery. 2023;**158**(10):1096-1102. DOI: 10.1001/jamasurg.2023.3211

[24] Ende V, Devas N, Zhang X, Yang J, Pryor AD. Internal hernia trends following gastric bypass surgery. Surgical Endoscopy. 2023;**37**(9):7183-7191. DOI: 10.1007/s00464-023-10206-7

[25] Raúl C, Jorge LL, Javier H, Claudia S, Yanette S, Diana T, et al. Complications of bariatric surgery. Internal hernia: A potentially fatal condition: A case report and review of the literature. Revista Colombiana Gastroenterologia [Internet]. 2007;**22**(3):243-248. Available from: http://www.scielo.org.co/scielo.php?script=sci_arttext&pid=S0120-99572007000300014&lng=en

[26] Altieri MS, Carter J, Aminian A, Docimo S Jr, Hinojosa MW, Cheguevara A, et al. Clinical issues Committee of the American Society for metabolic and bariatric surgery. American Society for Metabolic and Bariatric Surgery literature review on prevention, diagnosis, and management of internal hernias after roux-en-Y gastric bypass. Surgery for Obesity and Related Diseases. 2023;**19**(7):763-771. DOI: 10.1016/j.soard.2023.03.019

[27] Patel K, Serapiglia V, Rizzo AN, Varre J, Sonnanstine T. A paradoxical internal hernia at Brolin's anti-obstruction stitch following roux-en-Y gastric bypass: A case report. Journal of Surgical Case Reports. 2023;**2023**(10):rjad554. DOI: 10.1093/jscr/rjad554

[28] Bruinsma FFE, van der Burg SJC, El Adel S, Schouten R, Smeets SJM. Quality of stapled mesenteric defect closure influences the chance of reopening after laparoscopic roux-en-Y gastric bypass surgery. Updates in Surgery. 2024;**76**:1405-1412. DOI: 10.1007/s13304-024-01751-4

[29] Vilallonga R, Beisani M, Sanchez-Cordero S, Ruiz G, de Gordejuela A, Rodríguez-Luna MR, et al. Abdominal wall hernia and metabolic bariatric surgery. Journal of Laparoendoscopic & Advanced Surgical Techniques. Part A. 2020;**30**(8):891-895. DOI: 10.1089/lap.2020.0257

[30] Xu Z, Guo W. Clinical research progress of mesenteric internal hernia after roux-en-Y reconstruction. Zhonghua Wei Chang Wai Ke Za Zhi. 2017;**20**(3):352-356

[31] Apostolou KG, Lazaridis II, Kanavidis P, Triantafyllou M, Gkiala A, Alexandrou A, et al. Incidence and risk factors of symptomatic Petersen's hernias in bariatric and upper gastrointestinal surgery: A systematic review and meta-analysis. Langenbeck's Archives of Surgery. 2023;**408**(1):49. DOI: 10.1007/s00423-023-02798-4

[32] Lopera CA, Vergnaud JP, Cabrera LF, Sanchez S, Pedraza M, Vinck EE, et al. Preventative laparoscopic repair of Petersen's space following gastric bypass surgery reduces the incidence of Petersen's hernia: A comparative study. Hernia. 2018;**22**(6):1077-1081. DOI: 10.1007/s10029-018-1814-0

[33] Mahawar KK, Parmar C, Graham Y. One anastomosis gastric bypass: Key technical features, and prevention and management of procedure-specific complications. Minerva Chirurgica. 2019;**74**(2):126-136. DOI: 10.23736/S0026-4733.18.07844-6

[34] Geubbels N, Lijftogt N, Fiocco M, van Leersum NJ, Wouters MW, et al. Meta-analysis of internal herniation after gastric bypass surgery. The British Journal of Surgery. 2015;**102**(5):451-460. DOI: 10.1002/bjs.9738

[35] Stenberg E, Szabo E, Ågren G, Ottosson J, Marsk R, Lönroth H, et al. Closure of mesenteric defects in laparoscopic gastric bypass:

A multicenter, randomized, parallel, open-label trial. Lancet. 2016;**387**(10026):1397-1404. DOI: 10.1016/S0140-6736(15)01126-5

[36] Perim CA, Guedes MAE, Carvalho MFCE, Lopes PGF, Simões RL. A simple method for the diagnosis of Petersen's hernia compromising the biliopancreatic limb. Arquivos Brasileiros de Cirurgia Digestiva. 2019;**32**(1):e1429. DOI: 10.1590/0102-672020180001e1429

[37] El Nogoomi I, Nouh AK, Jaber AA, Toubah AM, Alkaram SS. Petersen's hernia after roux-en-Y gastric bypass: A case report. Cureus. 2023;**15**(12):e50757. DOI: 10.7759/cureus.50757

[38] Caixeiro L, Varanda J, Morais J, Ferreira A, Rios L. Petersen hernia after abdominoplasty: A provocative factor or a coincidence? Cureus. 2023;**15**(9):e45014. DOI: 10.7759/cureus.45014

[39] Fernández-Pacheco B, López-Tomassetti Fernández E, Hernández Hernández JR. Surgery and considerations for the repair of Petersen's space hernia after mini gastric bypass. Journal of Minimal Access Surgery. 2018;**14**(1):58-60. DOI: 10.4103/jmas.JMAS_133_17

[40] Calderón C, Castro A, Arciniega S. Petersen's hernia in a pregnant woman following roux-en-Y gastric bypass surgery: The importance of emergency surgical treatment. Cureus. 2024;**16**(3):e55815. DOI: 10.7759/cureus.55815

[41] Hernandez A, Petersen R. Laparoscopic Ventral Hernia Repair. The Surgical Clinics of North America. 2023;**103**(5):947-960. DOI: 10.1016/j.suc.2023.05.009

[42] Zhang Z, Miao L, Ren Z, Li Y. Robotic bariatric surgery for the obesity: A systematic review and meta-analysis. Surgical Endoscopy. 2021;**35**(6):2440-2456. DOI: 10.1007/s00464-020-08283-z

[43] Bertoni MV, Marengo M, Garofalo F, Volontè F, La Regina D, Gass M, et al. Robotic-assisted versus laparoscopic revisional bariatric surgery: A systematic review and meta-analysis on perioperative outcomes. Obesity Surgery. 2021;**31**(11):5022-5033. DOI: 10.1007/s11695-021-05668-4

[44] Nasser H, Munie S, Kindel TL, Gould JC, Higgins RM. Comparative analysis of robotic versus laparoscopic revisional bariatric surgery: Perioperative outcomes from the MBSAQIP database. Surgery for Obesity and Related Diseases. 2020;**16**(3):397-405. DOI: 10.1016/j.soard.2019.11.018

[45] Steenackers N, Brouwers E, Mertens A, et al. Late complications of biliopancreatic diversion in an elderly patient: A case report. BMC Geriatrics. 2021;**21**:631. DOI: 10.1186/s12877-021-02578-z

[46] Möller F, Hedberg J, Skogar M, et al. Long-term follow-up 15 years after duodenal switch or gastric bypass for extreme obesity: A randomized controlled trial. Obesity Surgery. 2023;**33**:2981-2990. DOI: 10.1007/s11695-023-06767-0

[47] Campanelli M, Bianciardi E, Benavoli D, Bagaglini G, Lisi G, Gentileschi P. Laparoscopic banded one anastomosis gastric bypass: A single-center series. Journal of Obesity. 2022;**2022**:4942052. DOI: 10.1155/2022/4942052

[48] Ospanov O, Yeleuov G, Fursov A, et al. A laparoscopic one anastomosis gastric bypass with wrapping versus nonwrapping fundus of the excluded part of the stomach to treat obese

patients (FundoRingOAGB trial): Study protocol for a randomized controlled trial. Trials. 2022;**23**:264. DOI: 10.1186/s13063-022-06252-6

[49] Nandipati KC, Bremer KC. Bariatric surgery emergencies in acute care surgery. The Surgical Clinics of North America. 2023;**103**(6):1113-1131. DOI: 10.1016/j.suc.2023.05.013

[50] Malaussena Z, Mhaskar R, Richmond N, Diab AF, Sujka J, DuCoin C, et al. Hernia repair in the bariatric patient: A systematic review and meta-analysis. Surgery for Obesity and Related Diseases. 2024;**20**(2):184-201. DOI: 10.1016/j.soard.2023.10.005

[51] Lazzati A, Nassif GB, Paolino L. Concomitant ventral hernia repair and bariatric surgery: A systematic review. Obesity Surgery. 2018;**28**(9):2949-2955. DOI: 10.1007/s11695-018-3366-x

[52] Karampinis I, Lion E, Grilli M, Hetjens S, Weiss C, Vassilev G, et al. Trocar site hernias in bariatric surgery-an underestimated issue: A qualitative systematic review and meta-analysis. Obesity Surgery. 2019;**29**(3):1049-1057. DOI: 10.1007/s11695-018-03687-2. Erratum in: Obes Surg. 2020 Jul;**30**(7):2860. DOI:10.1007/s11695-020-04592-3

[53] Oviedo JR, Hodges J, Nguyen-Lee J, Detz D, Oh M, Bombardelli J, et al. Robotic complex abdominal wall reconstruction: The evolution of component separation [Internet]. In: Hernia Surgery. London, UK: IntechOpen; 2022. DOI: 10.5772/intechopen.102001

Chapter 3

A Standardized Robotic Roux-en-Y Gastric Bypass

Pierre Blanc and Adel Abou-Mrad

Abstract

The reference treatment for obesity is surgery. Several approaches are possible, with the minimally invasive approach being the one recommended. This approach can now be performed with robot assistance. Bariatric surgery techniques are a succession of tips and tricks that the surgeon discovers as he gains experience. Robotic assistance adds further tips and tricks. The aim of this chapter is to give you the tips and tricks we have learned over the last 7 years and to enable every surgeon to read it and get help on a daily basis. This applies to all surgeons, experienced or not but also the nurses.

Keywords: bariatric surgery, robotic, technique, roux-en-Y gastric bypass, minimal invasive

1. Introduction

Roux-en-Y gastric bypass is the gold standard in bariatric surgery. It is a standardized technique, but there are many variations between surgical teams. We propose a robotic standardized technique to avoid undesirable effects, based on a literature review.

Despite its many advantages, robotic assistance is still being debated. Laparoscopy has been an advantage for patients but not for surgeons because, it is not at all ergonomic. The advantages of robotic surgery are for the surgical team: comfort, precision, and 3D vision. Hand-eye coordination is enhanced by 3D vision. There is no fulcrum effect, and at least the arms are fixed, so there is no pressure on the patient's abdominal wall. Bariatric surgery is a physical activity, as the abdomen is quite thick. This approach reduces the risk of musculoskeletal disorders for the surgeon and assistant. The advantage for the patient is less post-operative pain [1, 2].

2. Set up of the robotic program

Implementation of robot-assisted surgery requires a multidisciplinary approach, with appropriate training and cooperation of surgical, anesthetic, and technical staff.

3. Operating room configuration using the da Vinci X® system

3.1 Installation

The patient is positioned in the French position, with the left arm by the side of the body (**Figures 1–3**). The arms reach the head, the screen is at the patient's left shoulder, the console at the bottom right. We use five ports: 2 × 12-mm robots, 2 × 8-mm robots, 1 × 12-mm port with balloon for assistance (150 mm), and a Nathanson liver retractor to have a very good exposition. Three trocars are placed 18 cm from the xiphoid appendix before insufflation. The other two are placed a few centimeters lower. We use 100 mm robotic ports. The table is in 18° anti-trendelenburg position without any rotation. Assistant uses 45 cm laparoscopic instrumentation to avoid interference for assistant.

3.2 Suggested da Vinci® instruments

Arm 1: fenestrated bipolar forceps, Sureform®. *Arm 2*: endoscope 30°. *Arm 3*: Vesselsealer®, large needle driver, cissors. *Arm 4*: Cadiere forceps®.

3.3 Procedure steps for robotic roux-en-Y gastric by pass

The most delicate surgical steps are gastric dissection and the two anastomoses.

1. Division of the greater omentum

2. Inspection of Treitz angle and measurement of biliopancreatic limb

3. Closure of Pertersen's space

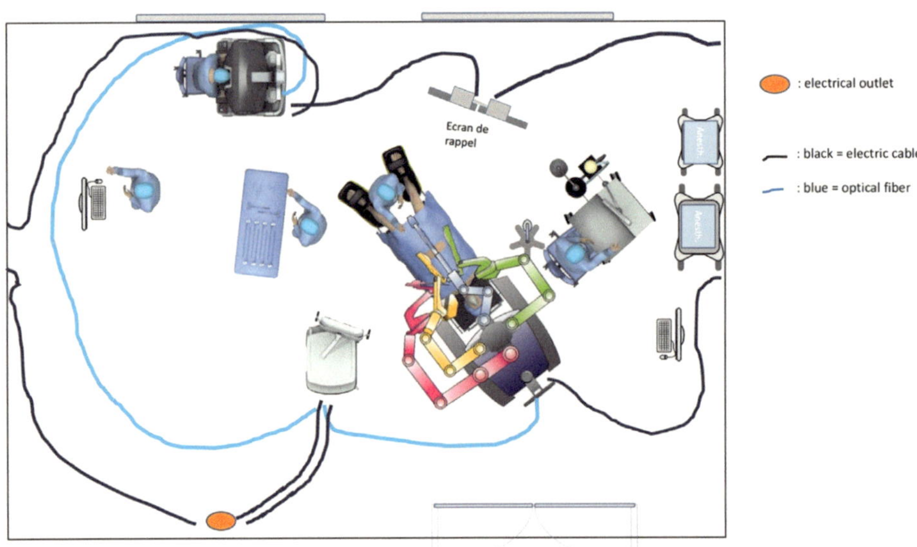

Figure 1.
Operating room setup using the da Vinci X® system.

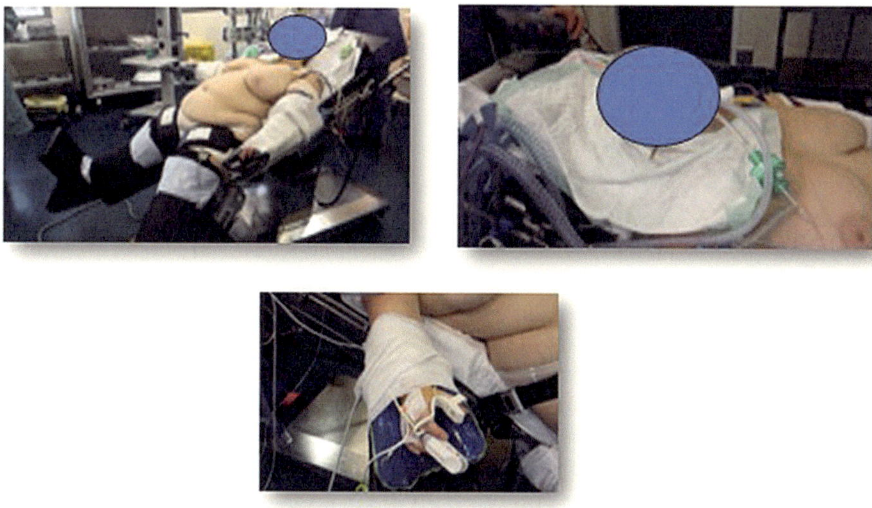

Figure 2.
18° anti-trendelenburg position.

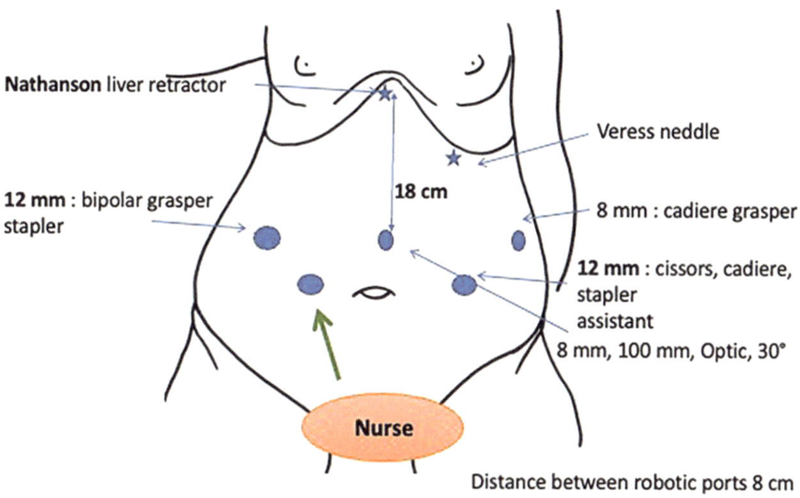

Figure 3.
Trocar placement.

4. Creation of the gastric pouch

5. Hand sewn gastro-jejunal anastomosis

6. Division of the small intestine

7. Measurement of alimentary limb

8. Second anastomosis

9. Mesenteric defect closure

10. Methylene blue +/- ICG test

3.3.1 Division of the greater omentum

Start the surgery by this division allows to test the installation, the instruments. Routine division of the greater omentum reduces post operative small bowel obstruction [3]. The exploration of Treitz angle and the Pertesen's space closure are easier after this.

3.3.2 Inspection of Treitz angle and measurement of biliopancreatic limb

Internal hernias, including left paraduodenal hernias, are rare and difficult to diagnose due to their non-specific symptoms and complex anatomical presentation. The presence of a paraduodenal hernia is a contraindication to gastric bypass surgery [4]. Correct identification of Treitz's angle helps to avoid incorrect assembly during surgery. Measuring at the outset allows good relaxation of the small intestine, and measurements are probably more accurate. Length measured between 75 cm and 100 cm.

3.3.3 Closure of Petersen space

Petersen space must be closed [5]. Sutures are easy with robot assistance. Doing it at the beginning, before the gastro jejunal anastomosis, is easier. We use non-absorbable and no barbed suture (15 cm, 26 mm needle).

3.3.4 Creation of the gastric pouch

The technique is the same as for laparoscopy, with much greater precision. This dissection can be performed with or without Vesselsealer®, which we recommend for revision surgery. The use of two 12 mm trocars makes horizontal and vertical stapling easier. We use Sureform®. Horizontal stapling is done with a 60 mm blue stapler. If the stapler does not pause during stapling, we switch to the white 60 mm feeder for vertical stapling. We compress for 10 seconds before stapling.

3.3.5 Hand sewn gastro-jejunal anastomosis

The advantages of manual anastomosis are fewer foreign bodies, less bleeding, termino-lateral anastomosis, possibility of making smaller gastric pouch. This reduces the risk of anastomotic ulcers and reflux and makes endoscopic exploration easier [6]. The robot makes hand-sewn anastomosis easier. Absorbable thread must be used. The correct length of thread is 15 cm, and the ideal needle size is 26 mm. The thread may or may not be notched. The hand sewn anastomosis is slightly more narrow to slow down the passage of food.

To avoid stenosis, the 38 Fr gastroplasty tube must be able to pass through the stomach opening, and it intubates the anastomosis until the end of surgery to calibrate and perform the blue test.

3.3.6 Division of the small intestine

Sectioning the intestine just after the first anastomosis facilitates the second and helps avoid Candy cane syndrome [7]. This section is performed with a 60 mm white cartridge.

3.3.7 Measurement of alimentary limb

The intestine is measured from 5 cm to 5 cm one grasper after the orther, always in the same direction. The length of the tip of the forceps used is 4 cm. The movement is counter-clockwise, one forceps after the other, with the wrists turned to the left. In the case of a history of abdominal surgery, this measurement is taken in number 2. Length measured between 120 and 150 cm [8].

3.3.8 Fashioning the jejunojejunostomy

The second jejuno-jejunal anastomosis is mechanical, to avoid a too narrow anastomosis. We use a 60 mm white charger placed in *arm 1*. This ensures good angulation of the anastomosis and avoids an acute angle between the alimentary limb and the biliopancreatic limb [9]. The closure is performed using barbed absorbable suture. With this technique, we avoid also the Candy cane syndrome.

3.3.9 Mesenteric defect closure

Closure of the mesentery defect is achieved using a non-barbed, non-absorbable suture [10]. The risk of the barbed suture is postoperative occlusion. The running suture is finished on the intestine. The aim is to achieve a harmonious anastomosis.

3.3.10 Methylene blue +/− ICG test

The blue test is systematic. It checks for leaks and stenosis. It is performed under pressure with 60 ml of gastric tube already in the small intestine. Blue can be paired with indocyanine green (ICG). It is also possible to check vascularization with an intravenous indocyanine green test using the robot's built-in Abilify technique. Intraluminal ICG presents a novel approach for detecting staple-line leaks in robotic bariatric surgery [11].

4. Closure and postoperative care

Trocars are removed under visual control. There is no drainage. The average duration of surgery is 2 hours.

The patient gets up and drinks the same evening. The next day, he eats a smooth 5-day mixed diet and is discharged on the first or second postoperative day.

5. Discussion

The role of robotic system in bariatric surgery is still unclear. The costs for the use of robotic system can be divided into three groups: the initial purchase, maintenance, and disposable parts. The surgeon has an action only on the disposable part, the operation times, and the complications. The arrival of competition will reduce costs. The development of this technology is still in its infancy. This technological evolution is inevitable.

6. Conclusion

Robot-assisted surgery offers the same advantages as minimally invasive surgery, with greater comfort for the surgical team and the patient. It is a reproducible technique. It is our preferred technique.

Author details

Pierre Blanc[1]* and Adel Abou-Mrad[2]

1 Clinique Chirurgicale Mutualiste, Centre Mutualiste de L'obésité, Saint-Etienne, France

2 Centre Hospitalier Régional, Orléans, France

*Address all correspondence to: pblanc@mutualite-loire.com

References

[1] Spiers A, J, Baillie S, Pipe TG, Asimakopolous G. Negating the fulcrum effect in manual laparoscopic surgery: Investigating skill acquisition with a haptic simulator. The International Journal of Medical Robotics + Computer Assisted Surgery: MRCAS. 2017;**13**(4). DOI: 10.1002/rcs.1837

[2] Tetteh E, Wang T, Kim JY, Smith T, Norasi H, Van Straaten MG, et al. Optimizing ergonomics during open, laparoscopic, and robotic-assisted surgery: A review of surgical ergonomics literature and development of educational illustrations. American Journal of Surgery. 2024;**235**:115551. DOI: 10.1016/j.amjsurg.2023.11.005

[3] Josefsson E, Ottosson J, Näslund I, Näslund E, Stenberg E. The effect of routine division of the greater omentum on small bowel obstruction after Roux-en-Y gastric bypass. Surgery for Obesity and Related Diseases. 2023;**19**(3):178-183. DOI: 10.1016/j.soard.2022.09.006

[4] Bhatta M, Katwal S, Paudel B. Left Para-duodenal hernia with distal bowel ischemia: An unusual presentation of the internal hernia: A case report and literature review. Radiology Case Reports. 2024;**20**(2):1165-1169. DOI: 10.1016/j.radcr.2024.11.005

[5] Vuagniaux A, Barberá-Carbonell B, Dayer A, Mantziari S, Suter M. Meticulous closure of mesenteric defects effectively reduces the incidence of internal hernia after laparoscopic roux-en-Y gastric bypass. Obesity Surgery. 2024;**34**(8):2806-2813. DOI: 10.1007/s11695-024-07306-1

[6] Feimster JW, Okorji L, Paul BA, Thompson KJ, Barbat S, Kuwada TS, et al. 10-Year outcomes of marginal ulcer formation and impact of gastrojejunostomy technique in Roux-en-Y gastric bypass. Surgery for Obesity and Related Diseases. 2024;**21**(4):412-416. DOI: 10.1016/j.soard.2024.10.039

[7] Celik NB, Cornejo J, Evans LA, Elli EF. Surgical management of candy cane syndrome after Roux-en-Y bypass. Surgery for Obesity and Related Diseases. 2024;**21**(5):554-558. DOI: 10.1016/j.soard.2024.11.006

[8] Cereser T, Heil J, Schöb O, Schlumpf R, Gantert WA, Infanger D, et al. Long-term weight loss of distal gastric bypass is moderately superior compared to proximal gastric bypass in patients with a BMI of 37-44 kg/m^2. Langenbeck's Archives of Surgery. 2024;**409**(1):162. DOI: 10.1007/s00423-024-03348-2

[9] Shi Y, Cao K, Wang ZJ, Han JG. Mechanisms and clinical management of small bowel obstruction caused by kinking of the jejunojejunal anastomosis after laparoscopic Roux-en-Y gastric bypass. Zhonghua Wai Ke Za Zhi. 2024;**62**(5):457-461. DOI: 10.3760/cma.j.cn112139-20231130-00247

[10] Aghajani E, Nergaard BJ, Leifson BG, Hedenbro J, Gislason H. The mesenteric defects in laparoscopic Roux-en-Y gastric bypass: 5 years follow-up of non-closure versus closure using the stapler technique. Surgical Endoscopy. 2017;**31**(9):3743-3748. DOI: 10.1007/s00464-017-5415-2

[11] Meng M, Saini J, Fan D, Singh A, Farkas DT. Use of indocyanine green to detect intraoperative staple-line leaks in robotic bariatric surgery: An observational cohort study. Cureus. 2024;**16**(3):e56991. DOI: 10.7759/cureus.56991

Chapter 4

Robotic One Anastomosis Gastric Bypass

António Albuquerque

Abstract

Robotic one-anastomosis gastric bypass (rOAGB) is an innovative bariatric surgical technique aimed at treating obesity and related metabolic disorders. This chapter provides an in-depth exploration of the procedure, focusing on its technical nuances, clinical benefits and potential complications. The robotic platform offers enhanced precision, improved visualization and greater surgeon ergonomics compared to laparoscopic approach. Key topics include patient selection, preoperative preparation, step-by-step surgical methodology and postoperative care. The chapter also examines outcomes such as weight loss, resolution of comorbidities and quality of life improvements, while addressing challenges like bile reflux and nutritional deficiencies. It highlights rOAGB's role in bariatric surgery.

Keywords: robotic one anastomosis gastric bypass, patient selection, preoperative preparation, step-by-step surgical methodology, postoperative care

1. Introduction

One anastomosis gastric bypass (OAGB) is currently the third most common weight loss procedure performed worldwide. It was conceived by Dr. Robert Rutledge in 1997 in the United States of America and named mini-gastric bypass (MGB). MGB was first reported by Rutledge et al. in 2001 with a biliopancreatic limb length of 200 cm, with good weight loss outcomes and a low complication rate [1]. In 2002, Dr. Miguel Carbajo in Spain initiated the OAGB variant of the MGB (the BAGUA—Bypass Gastrico de Una Anastomosis) [2]. This type of operation has gained proponents throughout the world, particularly increasing in the past years in Europe and Asia and has become one of the most commonly performed gastric bypass procedures in some countries. Although currently considered one of the most effective long-term bariatric-metabolic surgeries (BMS), through the years, there were "dark years" with the rejection of the procedure. With progressive popularity and acceptance by more groups and accumulating scientific publications, key events sequentially happened, which culminated with current approval by the world's most important Societies in BMS [3]. In recent years, combined restrictive and hypo-absorptive procedures have gained widespread acceptance and OAGB is a good example of a surgery that is balanced between simplicity of technical execution, low complication rates and good long-term results. When comparing the safety and efficacy between OAGB and other BMS, OAGB offers induced substantial weight and body mass index reduction, as well as substantial excess weight loss [4].

Moreover, it allows the resolution or improvement of all major associated medical illnesses and improvement in overall gastrointestinal quality of life [5]. Robotic surgery for bariatric surgery is a promising alternative to laparoscopic surgery, but the data are limited. The use of the surgical robot may offer special advantages for bariatric surgery and the first 50 cases of totally robotic OAGB/MGB were reported by Arun Prasad in India [6]. The robotic platform makes some of the steps of OAGB easier so that its standardization allows this surgical procedure to be performed safely and effectively.

2. Patient selection

Patient selection in OAGB is still a point of discussion among experts. There was consensus that OAGB is a suitable option in elderly patients, patients with low body mass index (BMI) (30–35 kg/m^2) with associated metabolic problems and patients with BMIs more than 50 kg/m^2 as one-stage procedure. Although can be a suitable procedure in patients with large hiatal hernia with concurrent hiatal hernia, it should not be offered to patients with grade C or D esophagitis or Barrett's metaplasia [7]. To ensure the best outcomes and minimize risks, patient selection involves careful consideration of multiple factors. Like any other patients to be considered for weight loss surgery, they must meet certain criteria based on the IFSO (International Federation for the Surgery of Obesity and Metabolic disease) guidelines. The patient selected to perform an rOAGB goes through a multidisciplinary approach, being evaluated for the fitness for the procedure by an endocrinologist, nutritionist, psychologist, gastroenterologist and anesthetist. In addition to the evaluation of the overall health status and the comorbid conditions, which must be stable and optimized before surgery, there are some anatomical and technical considerations that need to be addressed. After endoscopic evaluation, conditions like Barrett's esophagus, atrophic gastritis or intestinal metaplasia may influence suitability for OAGB and require other surgical options. Previous abdominal surgeries may affect the feasibility of OAGB and the robotic approach offers advantages in cases of adhesions or complex anatomy. Likewise, the robotic platform offers advantages in the approach to patients with super obesity, not only in terms of the mobility of the trocars and robotic instruments at the level of the abdominal wall but also by making it easier to deal with visceral fat.

3. Preoperative preparation

When considering any weight loss procedure, patients should be encouraged to lose weight prior to surgery to reduce liver size and the amount of visceral fat. This can be achieved through an integrated nutritional plan strategy, sometimes associated with anti-obesity drugs. The patient must continue taking medication to control comorbidities until the day of surgery and in cases of anticoagulant medication, a bridge to subcutaneous heparin should be made according to the anticoagulant drug used. There are no absolute or relative contra-indications for robotic surgery that are different than laparoscopic surgery. Prophylaxis of venous thromboembolism should be considered not only using sequential compression stockings but also through the administration of subcutaneous heparin. Prophylaxis of surgical site infection should be considered considering microorganisms in the upper gastrointestinal tract flora. After induction of anesthesia, it is necessary to introduce an orogastric tube to aspirate the gastric contents before the surgical procedure and to calibrate the gastric pouch.

4. Step-by-step surgical methodology

The preoperative planning for robotic surgery is consistent with other bariatric surgeries performed laparoscopically. The following procedure will be described using either a 4-armed da Vinci Xi or a da Vinci X. Successful robotic platform setup involves patient positioning, port placement and appropriate docking so that there are no conflicts between robotic arms. The choice of robotic surgical instruments may vary according to the surgeon's preferences, as well as the prioritization of the steps of the surgical procedure.

4.1 Positioning

The patient is positioned in reverse Trendelenburg. The patient's left arm should be placed alongside the body when using the daVinci Xi platform, since the patient cart is on the patient's left side, or both arms can be left open when using the da Vinci X, since in this case the patient cart is placed over the patient's head. In this case, because the patient's cart will be stationed above the patient's head, it is important that the anesthesiologist plans for easy airway and orogastric tube access. Whatever robotic platform is used, it is very important that the limbs rest over boards and restraint straps are used to safely position the patient for this procedure. The risks to a patient in this type of position include deep vein thrombosis, sliding and shearing, perineal nerve and tibial nerve. Padded footboards should be used to prevent the patient from sliding on the surgical table and reduce the potential for injury to the peroneal and tibial nerves from foot or ankle flexion. The reverse Trendelenburg can be accomplished with splitting legs. Split leg positioners provide midline access to the patient with independent controls for docking or hybrid steps of the procedure, if considered, like the small bowel measurement.

4.2 Port placement

Pneumoperitoneum is obtained by inserting a Veress needle in the left upper quadrant, below the costal margin on Palmer's point and the abdomen is inflated to a maximum pressure of 15 mmHg. When planning a bariatric procedure using a fourth-generation da Vinci platform (Xi or X), it is essential to respect the port placement so that they are aligned on a horizontal line located 20 cm from the target anatomy. Because the target anatomy for a rOAGB is the distal stomach, located slightly below the xiphoid, the camera port is placed 20 cm below the xiphoid 1 to 2 cm to the left of midline (**Figure 1**). The additional ports should be at least 8 cm from any adjacent ports. Robotic arm port 1 should be placed 8 cm to the right of camera port 2. Robotic arm port 3 should be placed 8 cm to the left of arm port 2 and arm port 4, 8 cm to the left of robotic arm port 3. The assistant port, if used, can be placed lateral to robotic arm port 1 (**Figure 2**). The main reason for placing this port lateral to robotic arm port 1 instead of placing it between arm ports 1 and 2 is that in rOAGB, it is necessary to obtain the maximum angulation of the laparoscopic stapler, when used, to allow a gastric section as transverse as possible of the lesser gastric curvature below the crow's foot. The assistant port can be placed between arm port 1 and arm port 2, which may facilitate the final gastric pouch stapling but make the first transversal stapling more difficult (**Figure 3**). The use of the assistant port may allow the introduction of swabs, sutures or other instruments if necessary. When not used, to use the robotic stapler, it is necessary to use

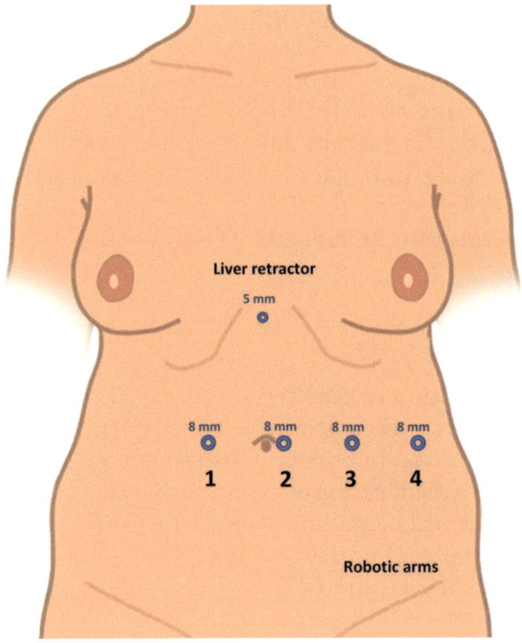

Figure 1.
Totally robotic one anastomosis gastric bypass port placement.

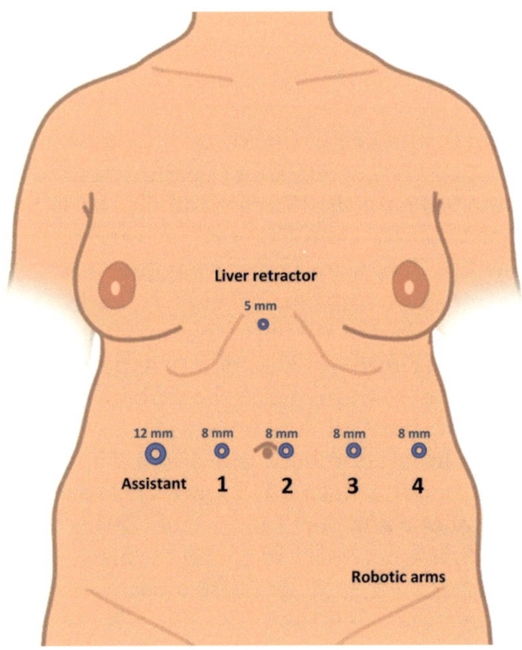

Figure 2.
Hybrid robotic one anastomosis gastric bypass port placement.

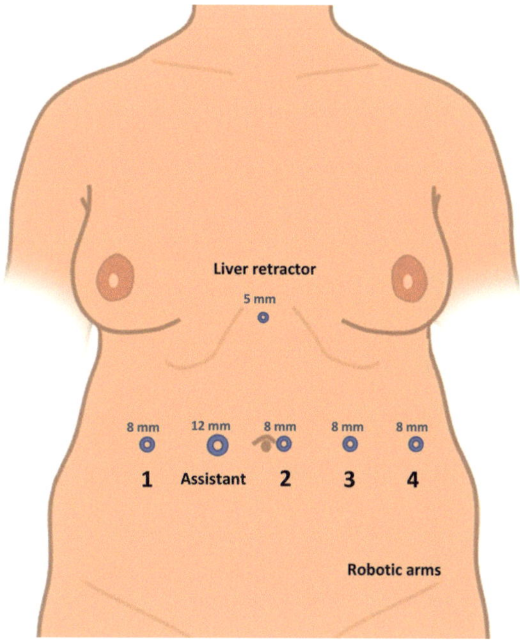

Figure 3.
Alternative hybrid robotic one anastomosis gastric bypass port placement.

a 12 mm cannula for robotic port arm 1 instead of the 8 mm cannulas used for arm ports 2, 3, and 4. An additional 5 mm port may be required to retract the liver using a Nathanson retractor in cases of hepatomegaly. However, the liver can be retracted using an intracorporeal suture between the diaphragm pillars and the anterior abdominal wall in cases of smaller livers and in exceptional cases, it may not even be necessary. Considering that the location of the ports follows certain specifications, it is imperative to perform adhesiolysis of any intra-abdominal adhesions to the anterior abdominal wall at the chosen port locations. Another type of adhesions, which make the surgical procedure itself difficult, are best treated with the use of the robotic platform.

4.3 Docking

Docking is commonly considered to be one of the factors that causes the greatest surgical delay when compared to conventional laparoscopic surgery. However, once the learning curve has been overcome, this phase does not substantially increase surgical time and correct docking avoids delays in subsequent surgical steps. Unlike robotic roux-en-Y gastric that requires to work in both the sub--diaphragmatic and infracolic compartments of the abdomen, meaning the need for a dual docking of the robot or a hybrid partial laparoscopic and partial robotic surgery, the rOAGB has the advantage of having all dissection and anastomosis in the supracolic compartment and is therefore it is a surgical procedure that is easier to perform using a robotic platform [6].

4.4 Instruments

The use of robotic instruments may vary according to the patient's specifications and the surgeon's preference. In most cases, although obese patients may have very large adipose tissue in the abdominal wall, long cannulas are not necessary. The vision equipment allows maximization of visualization using a 30-degree 8 mm camera. Endowrist® graspers such as Cadiére forceps®, fenestrated bipolar forceps or others with intermediate gripping strength such as Tip-up fenestrated grasper® can be used to manipulate the viscera. The Prograsp forceps® have too much gripping force, which can cause some gastric or small bowel injuries. The Endowrist® monopolar cautery instruments allow for careful and precise dissection and the use of monopolar curved scissors has the advantage over the permanent cautery hook in allowing cutting. Considering that large-caliber vessel ligation is not necessary to perform an rOAGB, advanced energy devices such as the Vessel Sealer®, Synchroseal® or ultrasonic energy are not usually used. EndoWrist® bipolar cautery instruments such as the fenestrated bipolar forceps or the Maryland bipolar forceps® allow most of the steps of the surgical technique. Performing an rOAGB involves creating a gastric pouch and a gastrojejunal anastomosis. For this purpose, it is necessary to use endoscopic staplers, which can either be those of the robotic platform, whose components are Sureform® stapler instruments with their respective Sureform® stapler reloads, or alternatively, the use of staplers used in conventional laparoscopy, through the assistant port. Gastrojejunal anastomosis can be manual with hand sewing or mechanical with a stapler. Suturing can be performed using any of the Endowrist® needle drivers. Usually, the large needle driver is sufficient, but if the surgeon prefers to cut the suture threads more quickly, the large suturecut needle driver can be used.

4.5 Procedure

OAGB consists of a gastric pouch between the esophagogastric junction and the crow's foot level, parallel to the lesser curvature, which is anastomosed laterolaterally to a jejunal loop 200 cm distal to the ligament of Treitz. Carbajo proposed the creation of even longer gastric reservoirs, of ≥20 cm, based proximally on the complete dissection of diaphragmatic crura and distally by entering the lesser sac halfway between pylorus and last antral branch of crow's foot (~ 2 – 2.5 cm from pylorus) [3]. The surgical procedure begins with the creation of a long, narrow gastric pouch, and to do so, it is necessary to open a window in the small omentum (**Figure 4**) below the crow's foot and dissect the phrenogastric ligament around the angle of His (**Figure 5**). Dissection in this area is best achieved with monopolar curved scissors or the cautery hook rather than with other types of instruments. Opening the window to access the small sac can be done by dissecting and isolating small vessels of the small omentum, ligating them with monopolar energy using monopolar curved scissors, fenestrated bipolar forceps or, rarely, using surgical advanced energy devices.

The gastric pouch of the OAGB is intentionally designed to be a non-obstructive conduit for food (like the esophagus) from its upper inlet to its outlet. The low-pressure pouch designed for this bypass procedure, must be created 1–2 cm distal to the crow's foot, to protect the esophagus from gastroesophageal reflux. To accomplish a narrow gastric pouch, the bougie size should be between 28 and 36 French. The gastric pouch should lie such that the medial aspect, the mesentery of the lesser curvature, points directly to the usual position of the ports to the patient's right and the neo-greater curvature (staple-line) points directly to the patient's left,

DOI: http://dx.doi.org/10.5772/intechopen.1009593

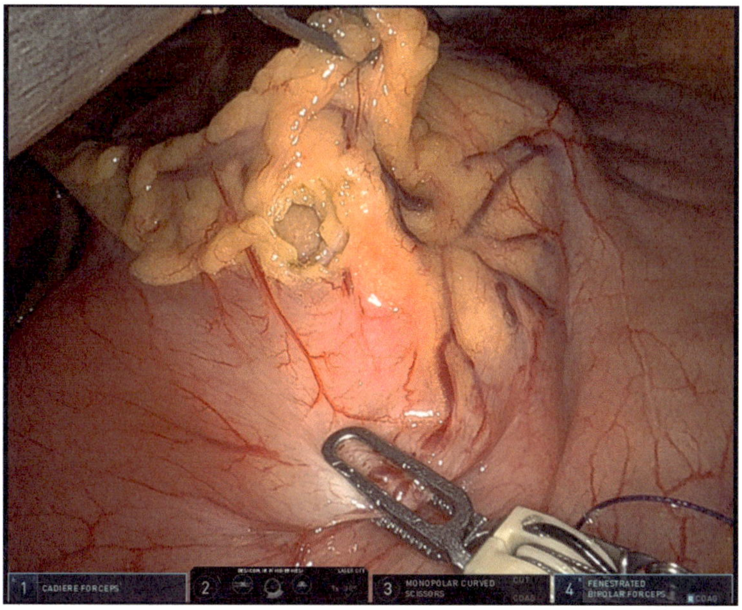

Figure 4.
Opening the lesser omentum below the crow's foot.

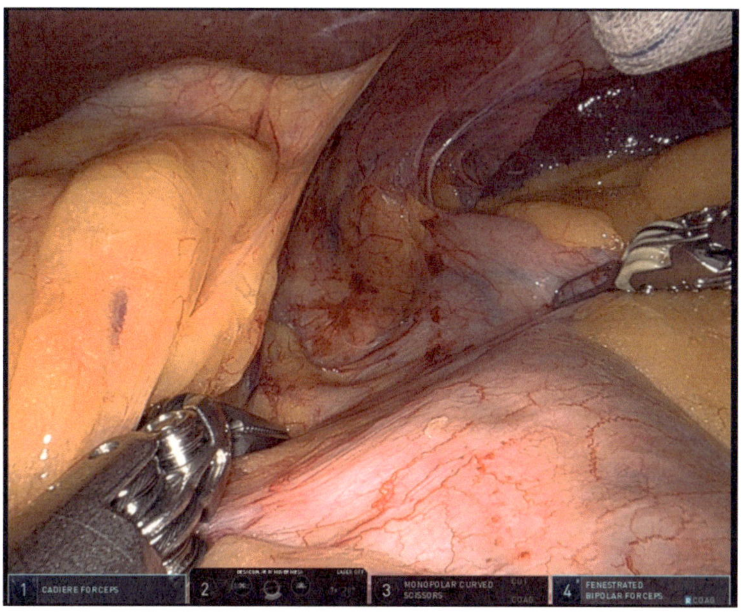

Figure 5.
Dissection of the phrenogastric ligament around the angle of His.

with anterior and posterior walls of the pouch being equal. In this way, the first stapling of the stomach must be perpendicular to the axis of the lesser curvature, using a 45 mm load (**Figure 6**) and the remaining vertical must follow a straight line parallel to the bougie, up to the angle of His (**Figures** 7 and **8**). For this vertical section, 60 mm loads should be used and chosen according to the thickness of the

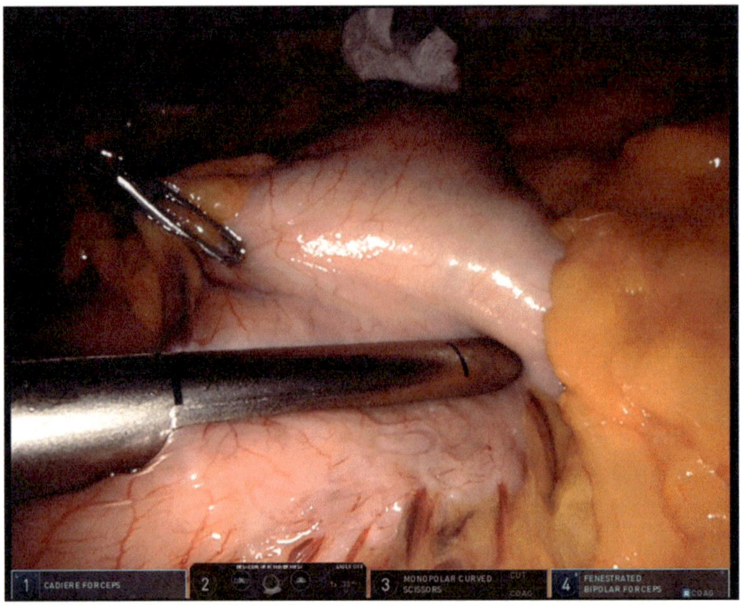

Figure 6.
First stapling of the stomach perpendicular to the axis of the lesser curvature.

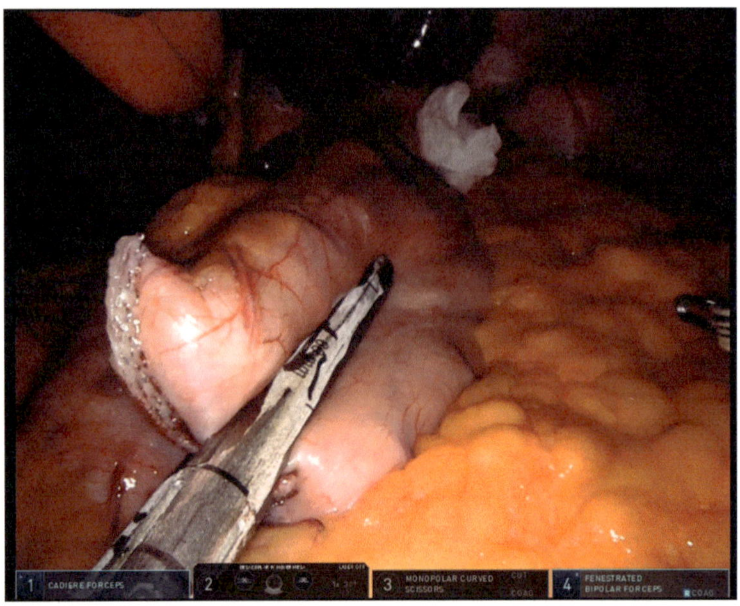

Figure 7.
Vertical stapling following a straight line parallel to the bougie.

gastric wall, greater in the antrum region and smaller as approaching the fundus. To create a gastric pouch with a straight vertical stapling line, it is essential to release any posterior adhesions that may exist between the posterior wall of the stomach and the pancreas. For this purpose, little or no energy may be required to minimize any burn injury to the gastric pouch. Once a long, narrow gastric pouch has been

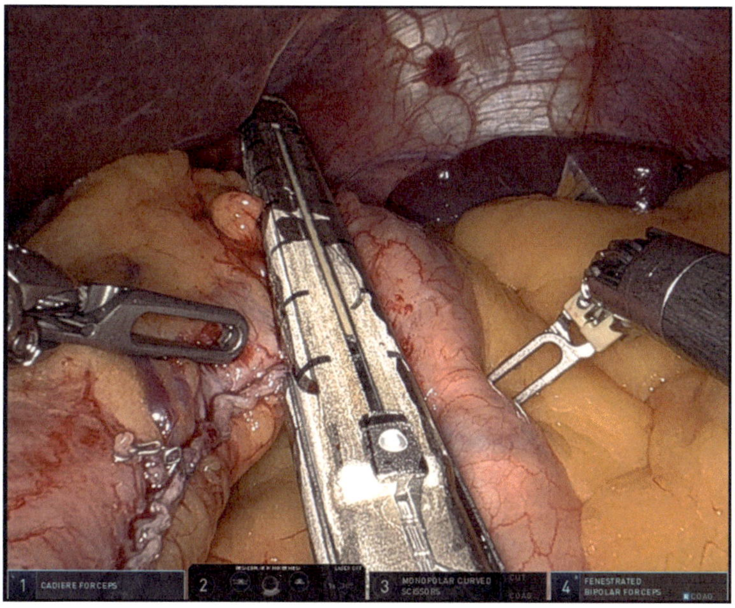

Figure 8.
Vertical stapling up to the angle of His.

created, the gastrojejunal anastomosis will be performed. Regarding technical standardization, there is no consensus on the minimum recommended length of the gastric pouch. Nevertheless, the position of gastro-enterostomy (anterior, posterior, on the staple line) does not make any difference to the outcomes, and the recommended length of the biliopancreatic limb must be 150 – 200 cm. The best way to choose the length of the biliopancreatic limb must be tailored as per the patient, and it is not mandatory to measure the total bowel length in all cases [8]. After identifying the site of the proposed anastomosis and the length of the biliopancreatic limb, prior to proceeding, it is advised to confirm that at least 2–3 m of the small bowel is present distal to the gastrojejunal anastomosis. But for this purpose, it is not necessary to run the entire small bowel. The gastrojejunal anastomosis can be performed manually or using a stapler. One of the advantages of the robotic platform is the greater range of movements that facilitates the execution of any intracorporeal suture. For this reason, some surgeons prefer to perform manual gastrojejunal anastomosis. However, its execution with a stapler (**Figure 9**), whether robotic or laparoscopic, entering through the assistant's port, is equally effective. In the latter case, it is necessary to close the joint gastrotomy and enterostomy orifice (**Figure 10**), for which suturing with the robotic platform is an added value. Whether performing a manual or mechanical anastomosis, it can be performed with any absorbable suture, 2.0 or 3.0, with monofilament or polyfilament material, in one or two layers. Although the safety of performing the gastrojejunal anastomosis using the robotic platform is high, it is recommended to confirm the absence of leaks with a methylene blue test. Despite being proposed by Carbajo, there does not appear to be any advantage or effectiveness of an anti-reflux stitch between the pouch and the afferent limb. However, although many surgeons believe that it is not always necessary to close the Petersen space, as it is a space created by the anatomical modification of the surgical procedure through which an internal

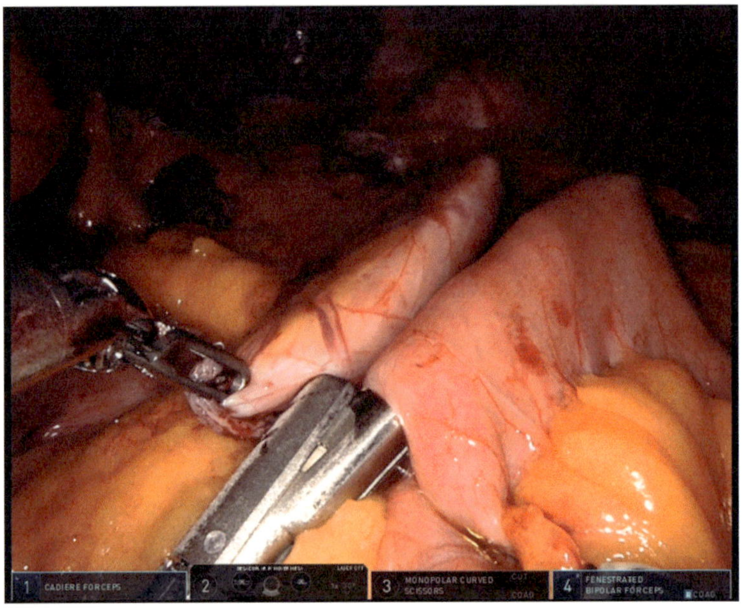

Figure 9.
Gastrojejunal anastomosis.

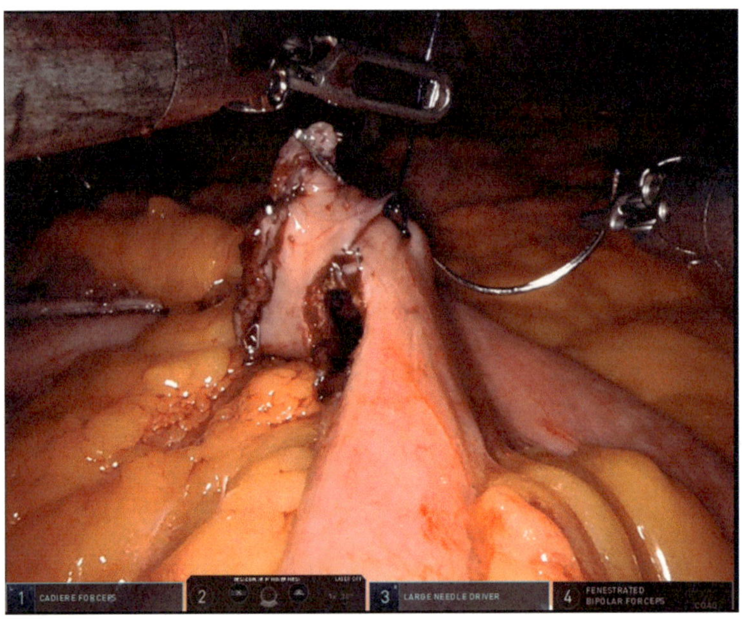

Figure 10.
Closing the joint gastrotomy and enterostomy orifice.

hernia with potentially catastrophic consequences may occur, it can be closed easily. Likewise, it is advisable to close the aponeurosis of the 12 mm ports, either by using a cannula for the robotic stapler or the assistant's port, whenever used. The same procedure is not necessary for 8 mm ports.

5. Tips and tricks

The following tips and tricks reflect personal experience in executing the steps outlined above. Regarding patient positioning, the option to keep the legs apart seems to facilitate a hybrid approach for small bowel measurement by laparoscopy or another surgical step prior to docking performed by laparoscopy, such as the release of intra-abdominal adhesions before the placement of the ports. Although some surgeons suggest a right-sided position of the operating table, there does not appear to be much advantage. What we consider essential is a pronounced reverse Trendelenburg to conveniently approach the angle of His and treat, if there is, any hiatal hernia. Placement of ports for minimally invasive surgery must be performed under direct visualization. Therefore, after blindly placing robotic arm port 2 for the camera, robotic arm port 4 should be placed first, further away from port 2, and then the camera should be inserted through this cannula and the insertion of robotic arm port 1 or any assistant port should be visualized. Finally, insert the camera through robotic arm port 1 to view the placement of port 3. When using an assistant port for stapling, considering that the creation of a long gastric pouch is one of the crucial aspects of OAGB, so that the first gastric section is as perpendicular as possible to the axis of the lesser curvature, it is important that it is placed laterally to the robotic arm 1. In addition to the perpendicularity of the first stapling, fewer conflicts are created when introducing medical devices through the assistant port and the robotic arms. However, due to the greater distance in relation to the region of the angle of His, in the last vertical stapling of the gastric pouch it is preferable to use a stapler with a long shaft. Closure of the aponeurosis of the 12 mm ports is recommended to minimize the risk of incisional hernias. A good strategy is to perform it right at the beginning of the procedure, not waiting until the end of the surgical intervention, when muscle relaxation is often suboptimal and may be more difficult. Therefore, medical devices can be used to allow the passage of suture threads for aponeurotic closure as soon as the 12 mm cannula is placed, tying the knot at the end of the intervention. One of the major barriers to robotic bariatric surgery is cost, so it is necessary to be selective and judicious regarding the use of surgical instruments. Most of the time it is possible to use only two graspers, a Cadiére forceps® and a fenestrated bipolar forceps, a monopolar curved scissors and a needle holder. The use of advanced energy devices is not necessary for most procedures. The sequence of the surgical steps varies depending on surgeons' preference. Some surgeons will begin laparoscopically by lifting the omentum and retract superiorly the mesocolon to expose the ligament of Treitz. The small bowel is run 200 cm to create a biliopancreatic limb. Before docking, it is recommended to evaluate the mobility of the omentum and mesocolon to decide whether the small bowel count can be done robotically or whether it is easier to do it by laparoscopy, a fact that may be an issue at the beginning of the learning curve. Our preference is to first measure the bowel and anchored to the omentum near the greater curvature of the stomach and then create the gastric pouch. When starting to create the gastric pouch, the window for entry into the lesser sac can be accomplished by ligating the small terminal branches with monopolar or bipolar energy. Care must be taken not to ligate too many vessels so as not to devascularize the gastric pouch. After the first transversal stapling to the axis of the lesser gastric curvature, the orogastric tube must be advanced and oriented to be parallel to the lesser curvature down to this level. Then vertical stapling begins, close to the orogastric tube, to create a narrow pouch. A tip that may be useful for creating the gastric pouch is to start by dissecting the area of the angle of His to expose the left pillar of the diaphragm and leave a gauze pad in that location. This gauze pad will serve as a guide when the stomach is being stapled vertically. Dissection of the angle of His should be just enough to create a window that allows stapling with the last reload. A very extensive dissection, particularly with division of the phrenogastric ligament over a large area, could break the physiological anti-reflux barriers. For this same reason, we do not find it necessary to remove the fat pad, especially because the compression of the staplers promotes effective crushing of this adipose tissue without compromising the quality and safety of the stapling. The cases in which an extensive dissection of the hiatal area must be carried out are when the existence of a hiatal hernia is suspected or previously known. Considering that medical stapling devices are safe, performing a manual anastomosis may take longer than with a stapler, in which the gastroenterostomy orifice where the stapler exits is smaller than the side-to-side gastrojejunal anastomosis itself. When the anastomosis is hand-sewed, it may be end to side, making the gastric pouch even longer. However, the main determinant of a long gastric pouch is the first gastric stapling being performed distal to the crow's foot. Our preference is to perform a stapled anastomosis on the anterior surface of the gastric pouch. One of the recommended precautions is that the anastomotic stapling is not too close to the vertical stapling of the gastric pouch to allow good vascularization of the gastric wall between the two stapling lines. Poorly vascularized gastric tissue can be the site of marginal ulcers, so whether on the posterior or anterior side of the gastric pouch, it is essential to achieve a well-vascularized margin between the two stapling lines. There is no consensus on the necessity of the anti-reflux stitch between the afferent loop and gastric pouch [8]. However, suturing the afferent loop to the gastric pouch with just one stitch is essential to remove tension from the distal anastomotic staple line (**Figure 11**). Although OAGB has a more distal gastrojejunal anastomosis, reducing anastomotic tension is essential to avoid dehiscence. In this sense, it may sometimes be necessary to open the omentum so that the loop of small intestine reaches the gastric pouch

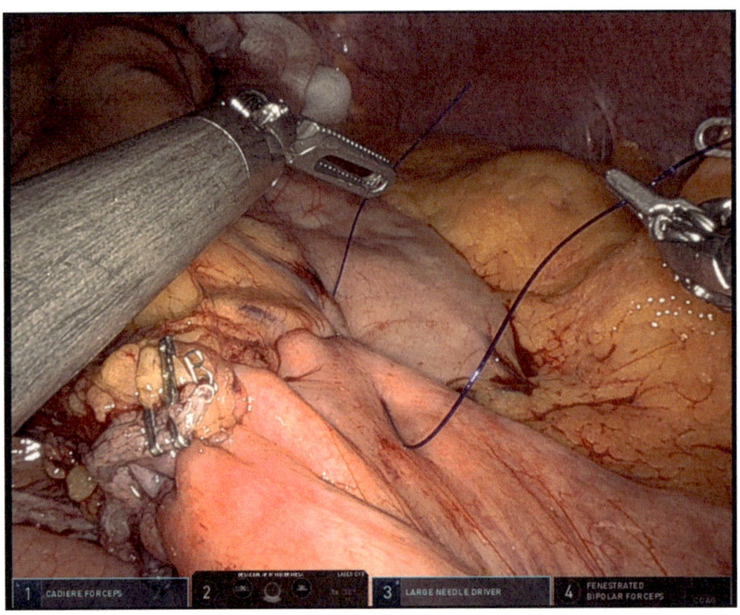

Figure 11.
Suturing the afferent loop to the gastric pouch.

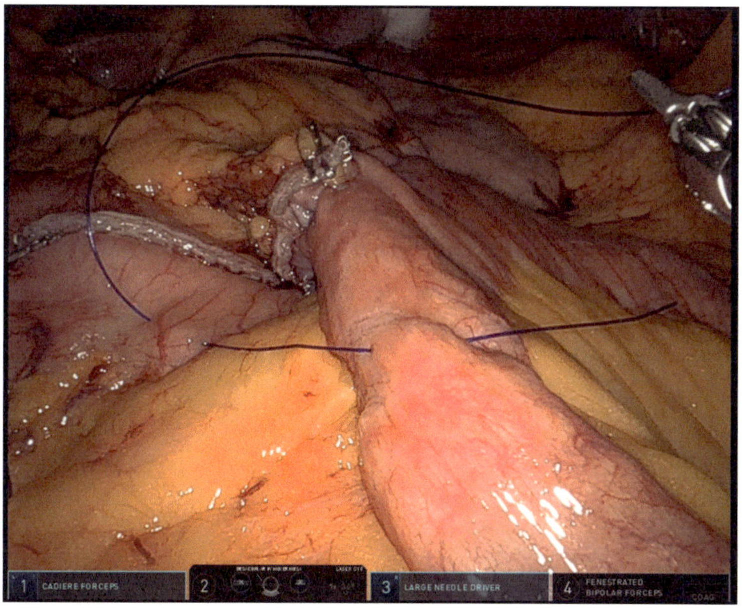

Figure 12.
Suturing the efferent loop to the excluded antrum.

without tension. Another important tip to reduce the possibility of reflux is to allow the post-anastomotic efferent loop to empty properly. To achieve this, it is important, in most cases, to suture the efferent loop to the excluded antrum with a stitch to avoid rotation and kinking of the gastrojejunostomy (**Figure 12**). To maximize the verticality of the efferent loop, it is recommended to apply cyanoacrylate glue between the efferent loop and the omentum, thus achieving good emptying of the efferent loop and minimizing reflux. Although many surgeons consider it unnecessary to close the Petersen space, as it is a space created by the anatomical alteration resulting from OAGB with potential complications such as strangulated internal hernia, it is recommended to close this space. There are several options for this, including suturing, which is facilitated using a robotic platform, or the application of cyanoacrylate glue, which, when using an assistant's port, can effectively allow good coaptation between the mesentery and the mesocolon (**Figure 13**).

6. Variations and technical modifications

The possible variations in a rOAGB involve modifications to the surgical technique itself and the use of the robotic system. As previously mentioned, there is a consensus that the gastric pouch should be long and narrow and that it is irrelevant whether the gastrojejunal anastomosis is performed on the anterior or posterior face of the gastric pouch or on the staple line. The technical aspect that is subject to the greatest variability concerns the site of choice in the small bowel for the anastomosis. The mini-gastric bypass reported by Rutledge et al. in 2001 has a biliopancreatic limb measuring 200 cm in length. However, the technique was later modified by Carbajo et al. and renamed one anastomosis gastric bypass. There are differences between both techniques regarding the gastric pouch and the anastomosis. For Rutledge, the

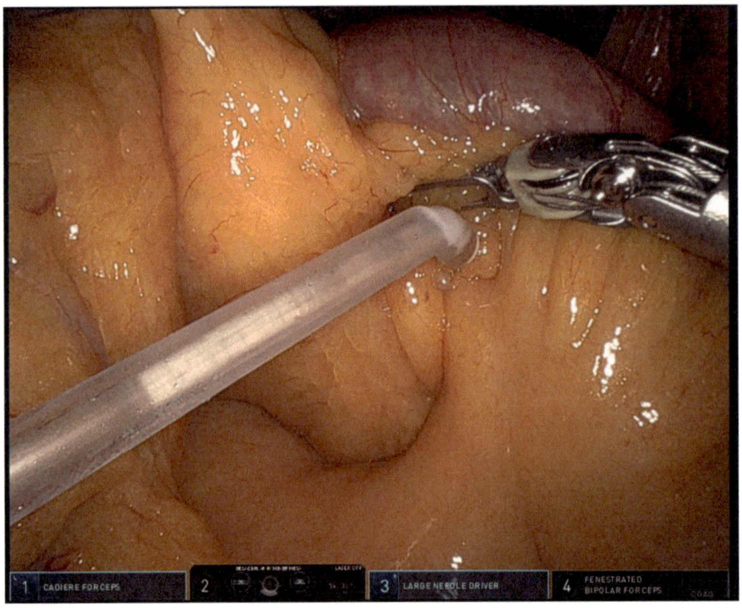

Figure 13.
Closing the Petersen space with cyanoacrylate glue.

gastric pouch should have a distal part that resembles the head of a snake, wider than in the OAGB. For Carbajo, suturing the gastric pouch to the afferent loop over a length of 10 cm is considered a technical modification that reduces reflux and is essential to measure the entire small bowel, with the chosen site for the anastomosis depending on a ratio of 60% of the total length of the small bowel for the biliopancreatic limb and 40% for the common limb. In rOAGB, it is worth noting that the option for a total small bowel measurement may be more easily achieved using a hybrid approach with this count being performed by laparoscopy. Although possible, the total small bowel measurement using the da Vinci X platform may involve redocking due to the need to change abdominal quadrants. The remaining variations concern the number of access ports to the abdominal cavity. In this sense, when a purely robotic technique is used, the four ports for the four robotic arms can be used, in which case a 12 mm cannula is required for the Sureform® stapler. In cases of a hybrid technique, the variations concern the positioning of the assistant port, as previously exemplified.

7. Postoperative care

Postoperative care follows the same pattern as laparoscopic bariatric surgery, which includes an enhanced recovery pathway with limited narcotics, a clear liquid diet and early ambulation [9]. Maintenance of IV fluids should be continued until the patient is tolerating a liquid diet and subcutaneous heparin should be continued postoperatively to minimize the risk of thromboembolism. Hospital discharge may occur on the first postoperative day, provided the patient is tolerating a liquid diet and there is no clinical suspicion of complications. No additional studies, such as laboratory or imaging tests, are necessary before the patient is discharged. Considering that long-term results are the main endpoint of surgical treatment for obesity and associated diseases, focusing on multidisciplinary follow-up is crucial to achieving weight reduction and improving comorbidities. For this reason, it is essential that the patient is committed to multidisciplinary follow-up, aiming not only at preventing but also at detecting complications. Two of the issues that are usually pointed out to the OAGB as disadvantages of adopting this surgical procedure are gastroesophageal reflux and nutritional deficiencies. Regarding gastroesophageal reflux, it is necessary to distinguish between acid reflux and bile reflux. To address the presence of which type of reflux, esophageal impedance, if justified, will be the complementary test with the greatest diagnostic accuracy. However, it is not usual, even in the presence of complaints, to request this test in the follow-up of patients undergoing OAGB. Although there is no consensus, even in the absence of complaints, it is recommended to perform an upper digestive endoscopy during the third year of follow-up. It is recommended that patients take proton pump inhibitors for about 6 months. Regarding the prevention of nutritional deficiencies, the focus should be on prevention, through multivitamin and mineral supplementation adapted to this bariatric and metabolic procedure, as well as early detection of deficits during outpatient endocrinology consultations.

8. Conclusions

The advantages of robotic surgery are common to all bariatric surgical procedures, such as better vision and precision of technical details, resulting in shorter recovery time and risk of complications. Within the scope of OAGB, the simplicity of the technique combined with the use of the robotic platform make rOAGB a safe, reproducible and easier technique to perform in cases of higher obesity classes and in the context of revision surgery. From the creation of the gastric pouch to the execution of the single anastomosis that characterizes this bariatric and metabolic procedure, all stages of this surgery are facilitated using the robotic system.

Acknowledgements

The authors are grateful to Sonia Realista for the illustrations.

Conflict of interest

The author declares no conflict of interest.

Author details

António Albuquerque
Curry Cabral Hospital, Cruz Vermelha Hospital, Lisbon, Portugal

*Address all correspondence to: amralbuquerque@gmail.com

References

[1] Rutledge R. The mini-gastric bypass: Experience with the first 1,274 cases. Obesity Surgery. 2001;**11**(3):276-280. DOI: 10.1381/096089201321336584

[2] Carbajo M. One-anastomosis gastric bypass by laparoscopy: Results of the first 209 patients. Obesity Surgery. 2005;**15**(3):398-404. DOI: 10.1381/0960892053576677

[3] Luque-de-León E. One anastomosis gastric bypass (OAGB): The story behind a name with 20 years of history. Obesity Surgery. 2023;**33**(3):956-958. DOI: 10.1007/s11695-023-06451-3

[4] Georgiadou D et al. Efficacy and safety of laparoscopic mini gastric bypass. A systematic review. Surgery for Obesity and Related Diseases. 2014;**10**(5):984-991. DOI: 10.1016/j.soard.2014.02.009

[5] Balamurugan G. Comparison of efficacy and safety between roux-en-Y gastric bypass (RYGB) vs one anastomosis gastric bypass (OAGB) vs single anastomosis Duodeno-ileal bypass with sleeve gastrectomy (SADI-S): A systematic review of bariatric and metabolic surgery. Obesity Surgery. 2023;**33**(7):2194-2209. DOI: 10.1007/s11695-023-06602-6

[6] Prasad A. Robotic one anastomosis (omega loop/mini) gastric bypass for morbid obesity. Journal of Robotic Surgery. 2014;**2014**(8):371-374. DOI: 10.1007/s11701-014-0480-1

[7] Kermansaravi M. Patient selection in one anastomosis/mini gastric bypass-an expert modified Delphi consensus. Obesity Surgery. 2022;**32**(8):2512-2524. DOI: 10.1007/s11695-022-06124-7

[8] Bhasker A. MGB-OAGB international club—Results of a modified Delphi consensus on controversies in OAGB. Obesity Surgery. 2024;**34**(12):4541-4554. DOI: 10.1007/s11695-024-07563-0

[9] Stenberg E. Guidelines for perioperative care in bariatric surgery: Enhanced recovery after surgery (ERAS) society recommendations: A 2021 update. World Journal of Surgery. 2022;**46**(4):729-751. DOI: 10.1007/s00268-021-06394-9

Chapter 5

Robotic Roux-en-Y Gastric Bypass: The French Orléans' Way

Adel Abou-Mrad, Miljana Vladimirov, Aman Goyal, Pierre Blanc, Sjaak Pouwels, Vikas Jain, Beniamino Pascotto, Luigi Marano and Rodolfo J. Oviedo

Abstract

Roux-en-Y gastric bypass is a gold-standard metabolic and bariatric surgery (MBS) procedure. The robotic approach is becoming more common. Surgeons adapt the technique according to their own style and experience. We describe step-by-step, with video links, the procedure routinely used in an expert high-volume French MBS center. This standardized procedure's presentation aims to facilitate surgery, reducing the operative console time and complications while harmonizing its practice. It helps the perioperative team staff in preparing for the procedure and demystifying the robotic use, to make their participation simple, harmonious, clear, and practical. Selecting simple robotic instruments and adapting the procedure to its simple aspects helps with diminishing its associated costs. This enables the surgeon and team to operate on a maximum number of patients with a fixed budget. "The French Orléans' Technique" is detailed. We consider it safe, feasible, reproducible, and easy to execute with a reduced learning curve. Once acquired, it enables moving to complex surgery. Economizing time and expensive instruments make the procedure affordable and closer in terms costs, if not equivalent, to laparoscopy. This chapter is a guide to resemble the usual companionship for surgical appraisal.

Keywords: bariatric, surgery, bariatric surgery, robotic, robotic bariatric surgery, obesity, by-pass, robotic by-pass

1. Introduction

Robotic Roux-en-Y Gastric Bypass (RRYGB) is a standardized surgical technique reported in 1969 by Mason [1] and has been practiced worldwide since. It is considered among the gold-standard metabolic and bariatric surgery (MBS) procedures [2]. The first laparoscopic RYGB procedure was presented in 1994 by Wittgrove and Clark [3]. In 2001, Horgan and Vanuno were among the first to report their robotic procedure experience as a safe alternative to laparoscopy [4].

Robotic RYGB is now routinely practiced worldwide [5]. The robotic approach is taking the lead. It is a feasible, safe, and reproducible technique. It is at least comparable to laparoscopy [6, 7]. Its learning curve is shorter [8, 9]. It is suitable for higher body mass index (BMI) [6], redo, and complex surgery [10].

In practice, there are as many specificities in RYGB techniques as there are surgeons, for they adapt it to their experience and personal perception of surgery.

This detailed description can help in becoming familiar with the robotic MBS approach.

Robotic RYGB can be considered the gold standard in patients without a history of previous MBS or digestive abdominal surgery.

2. Material

Since January 2014, over 4000 robotic procedures have been performed in the Centre Hospitalier Universitaire (CHU) d'Orléans—France. Nearly 800 have been RYGB procedures.

2.1 Establishing the robotics program

In December 2013, after a 1-day practicing course in a cadaver lab, a team composed of a surgeon, an anesthesiologist, and a scrub nurse went for a "case-observation" course in a pioneer French center at the University Hospital of Nancy in the Meuth-et-Moselle state—France. Two cases of robotic RYGB were performed using three arms of the Si da Vinci (Sunnyvale, CA, USA) device and counting two assistants and a scrub nurse at the bedside.

Back to Orleans, after debriefing, a specific lexicon is developed to coordinate the teams' gestures. The Si da-Vinci robot was deprived of a stapler device. The surgeon had to be patient and flexible enough to allow for the proper placement of the stapler by the assistant, a surgeon or a fellow, or the scrub nurse. The lexicon consisted of brief orders for stapling use such as "turn clockwise," "turn counterclockwise," "move to the right or left," and "bifurcate to the right or left." "Bifurcate" is meant to angulate the stapler in the proper direction. An ETHICON° Tri Staple 60 mm laparoscopic stapling device was used.

The first case was a robotic RYGB.

The technique was standardized with time, taking into consideration the stress status of the team facing a new technology. We have simplified it to the extreme and lower the cost correspondingly. We have stopped using the AirSeal° insufflator for patients with body mass index (BMI) less than 50, then after a while, completely.

The cheapest and simplest instruments have been chosen, avoiding expensive energy devices. The use of ultrasound dissectors was abandoned while favoring the bipolar forceps. A Cadiere forceps, a hook, and a needle driver (mega suture cut) were also chosen. Later, the robotic stapler was adopted with the acquisition of two da Vinci X devices.

This helped limit the cost and simplify the perioperative instrument trays, the material's storage, and the scrub nurse's burden.

3. Patient's management

At the first medical consultation, preoperative optimization takes at least 6 months, with multidisciplinary practitioners as recommended by the French High Authority of Health [11]. This includes the surgeon, the endocrinologist, the psychiatrist, the dietitian, the pulmonologist, the cardiologist, the gastroenterologist, and the

DOI: http://dx.doi.org/10.5772/intechopen.1010117

rheumatologist when needed. The gynecologist plays a key role in pregnancy prevention for about one and a half years after surgery. Infertility disorders with a desire for pregnancy are considered as added MBS surgical eligibility factor [11]. Urinary incontinence related to obesity is considered as another similar factor [11].

A specialized multidisciplinary commission states the acceptability of the patient's completed file. The surgical technique is chosen in accordance with the contraindications for sleeve gastrectomy (SG) such as severe GERD, esophagitis, Barrett's esophagus, hiatal hernia, or for RYGB including Crohn's disease, Biermer syndrome (if not

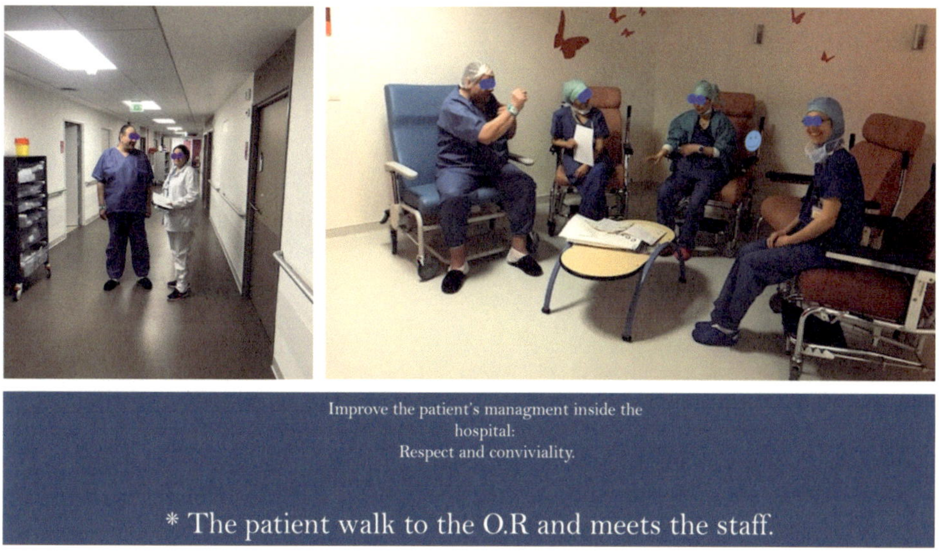

Figure 1.
Improve the patient's management inside the hospital: Respect and conviviality. The patient walk to the OR and meets the staff.

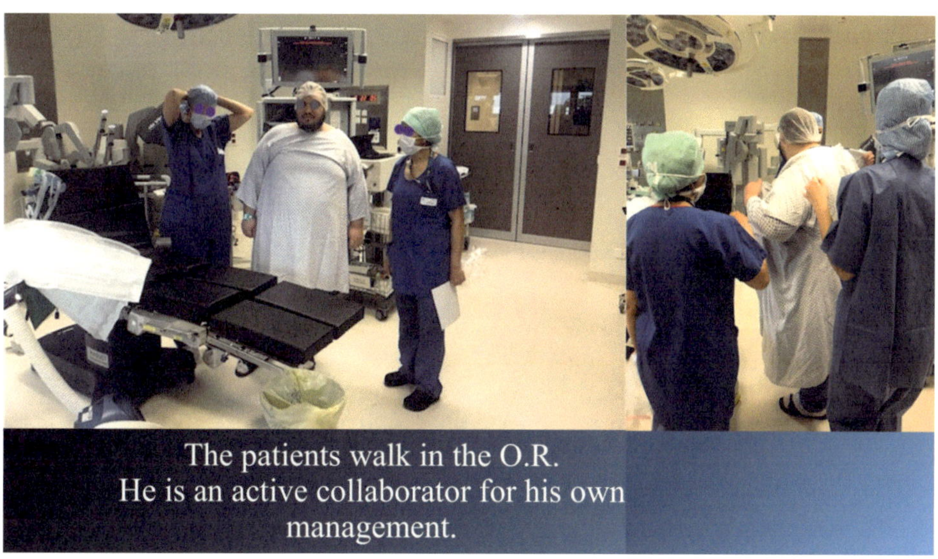

Figure 2.
The patients walk in the OR. He is an active collaborator for his own management.

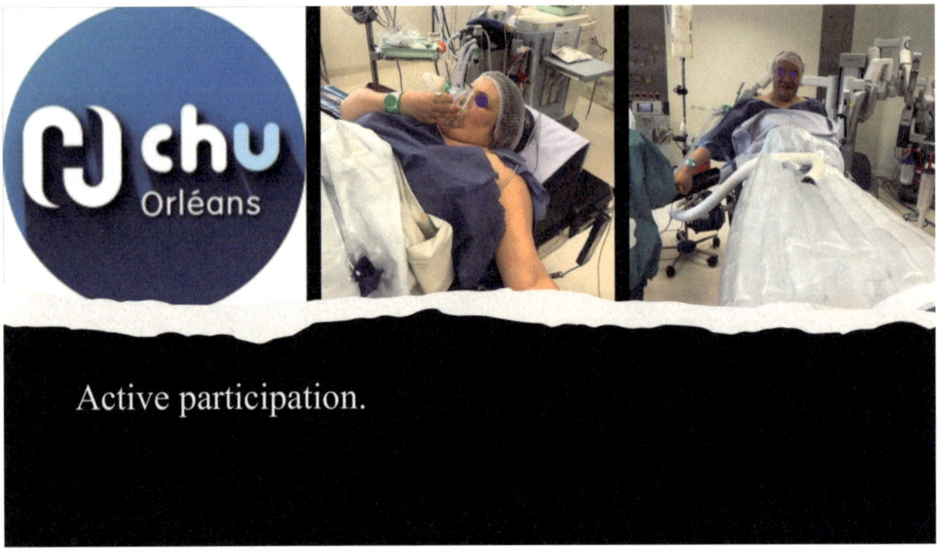

Figure 3.
Active participation.

associated with complementary gastric remnant resection in this last condition), and pathology or conditions with mandatory need to a permanent endoscopic access to the pylorus, duodenum, pancreas and biliary tract.

The patient is briefed about the type of surgery, potential complications, and short and long-term outcomes. After being fully informed and in the absence of specific contraindications, the patient chooses the preferred surgical technique. He is considered as an active collaborator for his own healthcare.

He is, usually, admitted on the morning of surgery, prepared, and accompanied to the operating theater, on foot, if possible. He is settled at the reception saloon and briefed by the surgical team.

The patients enter, the operating theater, on foot. They are welcomed in a dedicated space and briefed (**Figures 1–3**).

4. Anesthesia protocol

A specific opioid-free anesthetic protocol is considered (**Figure 1**). It is meant to avoid opioid fat-tissue accumulation, preventing potential postoperative secondary respiratory distress (**Table 1**).

5. Surgical settings

- The position on the operating table (Video 1, http://bit.ly/4lbSOyF):

The patient is in a flat position and at 15-degree reverse Trendelenburg tilt. The legs are stretched apart in the "French position." Intermittent pneumatic compression devices wrap the legs to prevent phlebitis. The left arm is kept aside from the patient's body. The right arm is in abduction-position allowing intravenous perfusions and anesthesia drugs' administration. The table is at 15-degree reverse Trendelenburg tilt.

- **Preparation of Dexdor syringe**

  1. *Main syringe:*

     One ampoule of 200 γ/2 mL of Dexdor diluted in 20 mL of 9% NaCl solution for a 10 γ/mL concentration

  2. *Load dose syringe:*

     20 γ/5 mL ⇒ 4 γ/mL

     (2 mL of the main syringe added to 3 mL of 9% NaCl)

     To be injected at the onset of peripheral vein perfusion, before anesthetic induction → 0.25 γ/kg (ideal weight, at a max of 20 γ)

  3. *Induction's syringe and ongoing perfusion:*

     Syringe of 50 mL of: 50 γ Dexdor (5 mL main syringe) + 50 mg of Ketamin (1 A of 5 mL) + 500 mg of Xylocain to be added in 50 mL of 9% NaCl

  4. *Speed of administration = 1/10th of the ideal weight (example: 60 kg = S6)*

- **Induction setting:**

  100 mL of 9% NaCl with 10 mg of Dexamethasone + 3 g of magnesium + 100 of Ketoprofen
  Intravenous anesthesia with concentration goal Propofol (think of installing the Bispectral (BIS) monitoring)
  Curare with neuromuscular transfer monitoring (NMT)

Table 1.
Protocol opioid free anesthesia (OFA).

- The X da Vinci° column's device is on the right side of the patient.
- Docking is cephalic.
- The trocars' placements are traced (Video 1, http://bit.ly/4lbSOyF). They are described further.
- 300 mg of Ropivacaïne (40 cc–7%) are injected on the intended trocars' sites before incision.
- Performing the pneumoperitoneum and the trocars' placement (Video 2, http://bit.ly/4lbSOyF):

Palmer/Veress needle is inserted through the tissues. A "water-drop" and "syringe air infusion and aspiration" tests are performed to confirm the intraperitoneal needle-tip's positioning.

- o The water-drop test:
- o The first 8 mm incision is made on a medial vertical line at 15 to 20 cm under the xyphoid process. The Palmer/Veress needle is held against the subcutaneous tissue. A drop of water is placed on the needle's edge. The needle is then pushed through. The drop goes inside the needle when the tip is in a negative pressure cavity. Going through the peritoneum is marked by a second click of the needle system. This indicates having entered the peritoneal cavity.
- o The "syringe air infusion and aspiration" tests:

- o A 20 cc syringe is used to inject and then aspirate air through the needle. If the injected air is withdrawn, the tip is in the abdominal wall or in a closed cavity or obliterated by tissues like the omentum. If not, the tip is in the abdominal cavity.

If blood or digestive liquid is obtained, an iatrogenic complication is ongoing, and the surgeon must react conforming with surgical experience.

If the tests fail, the soft tip mandril's 8 mm robotic trocar (no. 2) can be, carefully, used for a blunt intraabdominal introduction. It goes leftward on an oblique trajectory to avoid the ligamentum teres. Its intraabdominal position is visually controlled, before insufflation, ruling out eventual iatrogenic injuries.

CO_2 insufflation begins. The intraabdominal pressure is settled at 14 mmHg. The gas flow is settled at 40 mL/second.

A rapid visual exploration of the peritoneal cavity is made to rule out tissue injury.

With the camera in place (trocars no. 2), the other trocars are placed under direct vision. The robotic trocars are placed respecting a minimum of 8 cm distance between each. They are inserted from the farthest to the nearest.

If needed, and conforming with the surgeon's habit, a 12 mm single-use trocar is placed on the axillary line 5 cm below the right costal arc for a five-digit expandable liver retractor lifting and reclining the liver to the right, clearing the view to the perigastric upper field and the esophageal hiatus.

The second robotic 8 mm trocar (no. 1) is placed on a mid-clavicular vertical line, 3 cm under the right costal cartilage for the bipolar forceps.

A 12 mm single-use "assistant-trocar" is placed at 8 cm equidistance of the former two robotic trocars. It is used for suction, intraabdominal introduction and withdrawal of suture, and surgical-glue instillation.

The third 12 mm robotic trocar (no. 3) is placed at, nearly, 5 cm to the left of the umbilicus, 35 to 40 cm below the costal cartilage, on the midclavicular anterior vertical line. It is used for the robotic stapler, the hook, and the needle holder.

The Cadiere forceps' fourth 8 mm trocar (no. 4) is placed on the vertical mid-left axillary line below the costal arc by an equilateral triangulation with the nos. 2 and 3 trocars.

Once the trocars are placed, the robot (da Vinci X) is brought into a cephalic docking position. The robotic trocars are docked to its arms while avoiding arm collisions.

At the surgeon console, the surgeon visually controls the instruments, brought forth to their respective operating positions.

The monopolar electrosurgical power is settled on zero for cutting and 50 to 4 for coagulation. The bipolar forceps device is settled on 50 to 4.

6. The robotic RYGB procedure and technical aspects

6.1 The gastric pouch

An eventual hiatal hernia is ruled out or dealt with if present (see full gastric bypass procedure: Video 0, http://bit.ly/4lbSOyF).

A bougie of 36 French can be used to calibrate the pouch (Video 3, http://bit.ly/4lbSOyF).

A 2.5 cm wide and nearly 10 cm, which is longer than usual gastric pouch is made. It is believed to be less ulcerogenic compared to short ones due to better vascular preservation.

The His angle can be addressed primarily from above, or secondarily, if its retro gastric access seems difficult. The dissection is led with the hook, and hemostasis is mostly with the bipolar forceps. Hemostatic clips or resorbable 3-0 V-Lock running sutures can be applied on the stapler line when needed.

At the lower curve of the stomach, the dissection starts by lifting the stomach to a horizontal position and entering, close to the gastric wall, the retro gastric space between the second and third vascular pedicles. A tunnel is created perpendicularly to the lesser curve, enough to insert 4 to 5 cm of the stapler's thin jaw. Usually, a 60 cm blue Smart-Fire SureForm° cartridge is used. It is clamped for around 15 seconds before firing. This allows tissue flattening and hemostasis for optimal stapling. The cartridge is fired. Unfolded clips are thoroughly removed, avoiding tissue's tearing if stocked at the edge of the next cartridge's blade. The other cartridges are fired perpendicularly.

The bursa-omentalis is entered. The stapling is led toward the left triangular liver's ligament, creating a nearly 25 cm^2 pouch. More cartridges, blue or white depending on the tissue's thickness, are fired till separating the pouch from the remnant at 1 to 2 cm away to the left from the His angle. This is meant to avoid gastroesophageal stricture. The separation must be complete to avoid gastro-gastric fistulae-simulating residual passage.

Omentopexy can be done if the stapled left line of the pouch needs to be straightened or for hemostatic purposes.

A stay stitch is applied distally on the vertical stapled line of the pouch, one to one and a half cm close to its edge. It will be used for the back layer of the gastro-jejunal anastomosis.

6.2 The gastrojejunostomy end to side anastomosis

The ligament of Treitz is located under the mid-transverse colon and the inferior mesenteric vein (IMV) (Video 4, http://bit.ly/4lbSOyF). It is exposed by lifting to the right, without splitting the greater omentum. This can be rendered difficult in case of fragile prominent omentum or a redundant mega-dolichocolon. The proximal jejunum is run clockwise for nearly 60 to 70 cm visually estimated length. The right gastro-jejunal anastomotic edge is secured with the gastric stay stitch. The one-layer full-thickness posterior-row anastomotic running suture starts from left to right of the patient. This allows direct visual control, step-by-step, while progressing from "far to near." It is done with the viscera still closed. An identical string is applied, securing the left edge of the anastomosis. It will complete the anterior row. A 2-cm length opening is made with the hook, successively on the anterior aspect of the gastric pouch's edge and then the jejunal limb. The anterior row starts with securing the left edge of the anastomosis by applying a U-shaped stitch, taking the back row, and then going to the other side of the stomach, as shown in the video. A one-layer full thickness or inverted running suture completes the anastomosis. The right edge is secured by an in-out-out-in horizontal U-shaped stitch applied on the bowel side, which is believed to close this part. The two strings are crossed anteriorly to favor strings' holding-in. Epiploplasty can be made in case of swelling or fragile tissues.

6.3 The jejunojejunostomy anastomosis: "The Special Abou-Mrad Procedure"

The efferent intestinal limb is carefully run counterclockwise for 120 to 160 cm, considering the BMI's severity (Video 5a and 5b, http://bit.ly/4lbSOyF). Any serosa iatrogenic injury is treated promptly by a stitch or applying a clip.

A side-to-side jejunojejunostomy, double way, double length, stapled anastomosis starts by applying a "specially prepared, called the magic one," traction 3-0 resorbable V-Lock string close to the mesenteric aspect, joining the two limbs on nearly 10 cm length. It is meant to induce large bowel adhesions believed to reduce introsusception (Video 5b, http://bit.ly/4lbSOyF: a revision case with exploration of the jejuna-jejunal anastomosis, many years after the RRYGBP, showing the length of the adhesion between the two limbs). The string is used to orient the joined limbs' axis to allow for the stapler's proper insertion. An opening is hook-made on the mid-antimesenteric aspect of the juxtaposed limbs to insert a 6 cm vascular robotic stapler distally and then proximally to create the anastomosis. A thorough control of the anastomotic intraluminal stapler line rules out bleeding or an eventual residual posterior gap. If needed, hemostatic running suture or clips can be applied.

The mid-anastomotic opening is closed with a running suture or a vascular stapler cartridge fired perpendicularly to the anastomosis axis in a pyloroplasty-like technique.

The two traction-string edge-anchor points are controlled, looking for potential breach.

6.4 Closing the mesenteric gaps

Closing the mesenteric gaps is mandatory to prevent small bowel obstruction [12] (Video 6, http://bit.ly/4lbSOyF). Preferentially non-absorbable suture is used or surgical glue.

Non-absorbable 0/3 V-Lock string was used early 2014. Then, surgical glue (Ifabond° 1 mL) was favored. Properly used, it is easier to apply, timesaving with less immediate and secondary complications such as mesenteric hematoma, occlusive plication of the floppy alimentary limb induced by the stitches, and mesenteric shrinkage [13]. It is, drop by drop, carefully instilled on dried tissues through a specific cannula. Sufficient time must be allowed to dry.

The mesenteric defect is closed. The distal alimentary limb is also glued to its mesentera, on its last 10 cm close to the anastomosis, to lay on it respecting an harmonious curve while avoiding floppy-kinking and intestinal functional obstruction.

The Petersen defect is closed by lifting the omentum and bringing together the mesocolon glued to the proximal alimentary limb's mesentery.

6.5 Splitting the afferent limb

The afferent limb is reached 2 cm close to the gastro-jejunal anastomosis (Video 7, http://bit.ly/4lbSOyF). The mesentery is entered close to the bowel and a vascular cartridge is applied by splitting the bowel and establishing the Roux-en-Y configuration.

A visual general field control is made. Hemostasis is secured. The liver retractor is withdrawn as well as robotic instruments.

The procedure ends by undocking the robot's arms, exsufflation of the abdominal gas, and closing the wounds by a subcutaneous resorbable monofilament simple stitch's string. We do not close the aponeurosis for the trocars are inserted with an oblique abdominal wall path that is believed to prevent incisional herniation. Specific surgical glue is applied as a wound dressing.

7. Postoperative course

After recovering in the postoperative suveillance area, the patient is transferred to the regular digestive surgical department.

Oral intake is allowed upon complete anesthesia recovery in case of the absence of nausea, vomiting, tachycardia, abdominal pain, or hyperthermia. The patient is thoroughly briefed. The diet begins with normal, consistent small pieces of food, taken in little quantities and must be carefully chewed until pureed consistency is achieved. Near 30 seconds are to be considered between each mouthful. No liquid is to be taken with meals. Aversion of fast-absorbed sugar, and sparkling liquid are to be considered lifelong. No edulcorate is allowed. The patient must favor slow-absorbed sugar aliments such whole meal bread, dough, rice and starch. The patient should eat in a standardized portion-controlled dessert's dish while avoiding refilling it with food.

If the diet is tolerated, the dietitian is consulted, and the patient is discharged on postoperative day 1, with specific written recommendations.

In case of emergency, the patient is instructed to call the emergency phone number provided and/or to urgently come back to the hospital if needed.

8. Conclusion

In our experience, the robotic approach allows for early oral intake, regain of physical autonomy, and quicker hospital discharge. The described French Orléans technique has helped our surgical team to be more efficient. Its set-up binds the team and facilitates perioperative management. It has been disseminated and taught to French and other European colleagues while enabling the establishment and proliferation of successful and safer robotic surgery programs. A further comparison with additional studies is needed to confirm its impact.

Author details

Adel Abou-Mrad[1*], Miljana Vladimirov[2], Aman Goyal[3,4], Pierre Blanc[5], Sjaak Pouwels[6,7], Vikas Jain[8], Beniamino Pascotto[9], Luigi Marano[10,11] and Rodolfo J. Oviedo[12,13,14]

1 Centre Hospitalier Universitaire d'Orléans, Loiret, France

2 Department of General and Visceral Surgery, Bielefeld University, Germany

3 Department of General Surgery, Mahatma Gandhi Medical College and Research Institute, Puducherry, India

4 Department of Surgery, Adesh Institute of Medical Sciences and Research, Bathinda, Punjab, India

5 Clinique Chirurgicale Mutualiste de Saint-Etienne, Centre Mutualiste de l'Obésité de, Saint-Etienne, France

6 Department of Surgery, Marien Hospital Herne, University Hospital of Ruhr University Bochum, Herne, NRW, Germany

7 Department of Intensive Care Medicine, Elisabeth-Tweesteden Hospital, Tilburg, The Netherlands

8 Department of Surgical Oncology and Robotic Services, HCG Manavata Cancer Center, Nashik, India

9 Department of General and Minimally Invasive Surgery (Laparoscopy and Robotic), Centre Hospitalier de Luxembourg, Luxembourg, Luxembourg

10 Department of Medicine, Academy of Applied Medical and Social Sciences-AMiSNS: Akademia Medycznych I Spolecznych Nauk Stosowanych, Poland

11 Department of General Surgery and Surgical Oncology, "Saint Wojciech" Hospital, "Nicolaus Copernicus" Health Center, Poland

12 Department of Surgery, Nacogdoches Medical Center Nacogdoches, Texas, USA

13 Tilman J. Fertitta Family College of Medicine, University of Houston, Houston, Texas, USA

14 Sam Houston State University College of Osteopathic Medicine, Conroe, Texas, USA

*Address all correspondence to: adel.abou-mrad@orange.fr

References

[1] Mason EE, Ito C. Gastric bypass [archive]. Annals of Surgery. 1969;**170**:329-339

[2] Maclellan WC, Johnson JM. Laparoscopic gastric bypass: Still the gold standard? The Surgical Clinics of North America. 2021;**101**(2):161-175. DOI: 10.1016/j.suc.2020.12.013

[3] Seeras K, Philip K, Baldwin DL, Prakash S. StatPearls [Internet]. Treasure Island (FL): StatPearls Publishing; 2024. 2023 Sep 4. Bookshelf ID: NBK518968. Available from: https://pubmed.ncbi.nlm.nih.gov/?term=Seeras+K&cauthor_id=30085510

[4] Horgan S, Vanuno D. Robots in laparoscopic surgery. Journal of Laparoendoscopic & Advanced Surgical Techniques. Part A. 2001;**11**(6):415-419. DOI: 10.1089/10926420152761950

[5] Morrell ALG, Morrell-Junior AC, Morrell AG, Mendes JMF, Morrell AC. Robotic Roux-en-Y gastric bypass: Surgical technique and short-term experience from 329 cases. Revista do Colégio Brasileiro de Cirurgiões. 2021;**48**:e20212982. DOI: 10.1590/0100-6991e-20212982

[6] Senellart P, Saint-Jalmes G, Mfam WS, et al. Laparoscopic versus full robotic Roux-en-Y gastric bypass: Retrospective, single-center study of the feasibility and short-term results. Journal of Robotic Surgery. 2020;**14**:291-296. DOI: 10.1007/s11701-019-00976-5

[7] Li K, Zou J, Tang J, Di J, Han X, Zhang P. Robotic versus laparoscopic bariatric surgery: A systematic review and meta-analysis. Obesity Surgery. 2016;**26**(12):3031-3044. DOI: 10.1007/s11695-016-2408-5

[8] Hirri F, Pickering OJ, Carter NC, van Boxel GI, Pucher PH. Learning curves for adoption of robotic bariatric surgery: A systematic review of safety, efficiency and clinical outcomes. Journal of Robotic Surgery. 2024;**18**(1):349. DOI: 10.1007/s11701-024-02100-8

[9] Bustos R, Mangano A, Gheza F, Chen L, Aguiluz-Cornejo G, Gangemi A, et al. Robotic-assisted Roux-en-Y gastric bypass: Learning curve assessment using cumulative sum and literature review. Bariatric Surgical Practice and Patient Care. 2019;**14**(3):95-101. DOI: 10.1089/bari.2018.0042. Epub 2019 Sep 24

[10] Vanetta C, Dreifuss NH, Schlottmann F, Mangano A, Cubisino A, Valle V, et al. Current status of robot-assisted revisional bariatric surgery. Journal of Clinical Medicine. 2022;**11**(7):1820. DOI: 10.3390/jcm11071820

[11] Haute Autorité de Santé. Guide du Parcours de Soins: Surpoids et Obésité de L'adulte. Saint-Denis La Plaine: HAS; 2024

[12] Sundbom M, Näslund I, Ottosson J, Stenberg E, Näslund E. Results from the Scandinavian obesity surgery registry: A narrative review. Obesity Reviews. Feb 2024;**25**(2). DOI: 10.1111/obr.13662. [Epub 2023 Nov 14]

[13] Stenberg E et al. Closure of mesenteric defects in laparoscopic gastric bypass: A multicentre, randomised, parallel, open-label trial. The Lancet;**387**(10026):1397-1404

Section 3

Hepatobiliary and Pancreatic Surgery

Chapter 6

Choledocholithiasis: Then vs. Now

Raghav Bansal, Palak Kirti Jain, Abhirami Babu, Vedant Sachin Kasmalkar and Samridhi Mahajan

Abstract

This chapter provides a comprehensive overview of choledocholithiasis (common bile duct stones), focusing on its introduction, etiology, pathogenesis, epidemiology, clinical presentation, and diagnostic modalities. With the evolution of treatment strategies, it highlights the paradigm shift in managing choledocholithiasis, particularly the growing preference for laparoscopic common bile duct exploration (LCBDE) over endoscopic retrograde cholangiopancreatography (ERCP). While ERCP has long been the standard of care, its limitations seen in failed or complex cases have catalyzed the adoption of LCBDE, especially in regions where advanced ERCP resources are limited. Further, it delves into the emerging trends, emphasizing LCBDE's advantages as a single-stage, cost-effective approach that reduces the need for multiple interventions and addresses challenges raised by ductal clearance. It examines regional variations in the adoption of treatment modalities, with LCBDE being more prevalent in the Indian subcontinent due to unique demographic and healthcare system constraints. Furthermore, the chapter critically evaluates procedural outcomes, patient safety, and the role of technological advancements—such as laparoscopic ultrasound and robotic assistance—in enhancing surgical precision and efficacy. By presenting evidence-based insights and practical considerations, this chapter aligns with the broader theme of advancing surgical education and innovation, as explored in Upper Gastrointestinal Surgery – Contemporary Techniques and Training. It aims to equip surgeons, trainees, and multidisciplinary teams with the knowledge and tools necessary to harness modern techniques like LCBDE for optimal patient outcomes. Ultimately, the chapter underscores how emerging trends in choledocholithiasis management reflect a commitment to improving procedural efficiency, minimizing complications, and addressing the evolving challenges in global healthcare.

Keywords: choledocholithiasis, common bile duct, pathogenesis, clinical presentations, laparoscopic common bile duct exploration, endoscopic retrograde cholangiopancreatography

1. Introduction

Choledocholithiasis is defined as the presence of gallstones (choleliths) within the common bile duct (CBD). The term choledocholithiasis is derived from the Latin word choledoco, meaning CBD, and the word lithiasis, meaning stones [1].

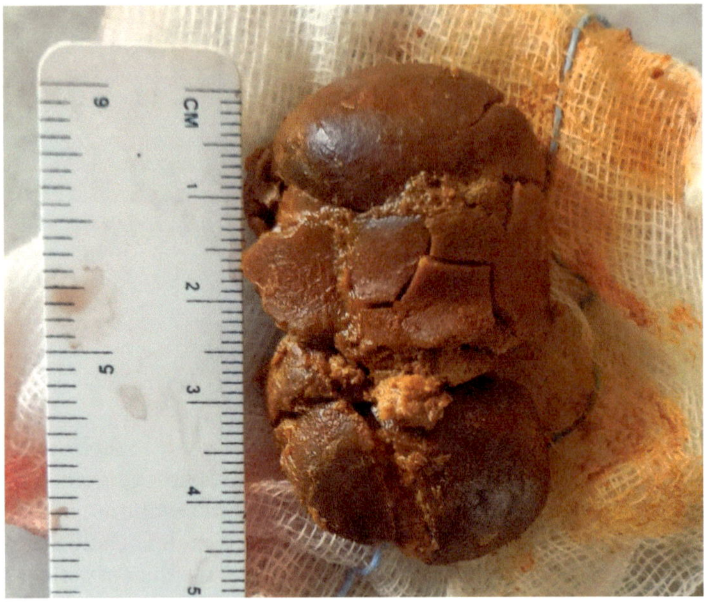

Figure 1.
A retrieved common bile duct stone through open choledochotomy.

Choleliths are typically formed when substances in bile, like cholesterol, bilirubin, and bile salts, are supersaturated and lead to nucleation, defined as the initial stage of gallstone formation where tiny cholesterol crystals begin to form within the bile in the gallbladder. These crystals gradually grow into stones inside the gallbladder. While smaller stones are easily able to pass through the CBD without causing obstructions, often stones larger than the diameter of the CBD (>5 mm) (**Figure 1**) result in obstruction—subsequently leading to further complications such as acute pancreatitis, cholangitis, jaundice, and sepsis [2, 3].

This chapter discusses the etiopathology of choledocholithiasis, diving into the details of the formation of choleliths, and highlighting the differences between primary and secondary choledocholithiasis, the risk factors involved, and common complications that arise as a result. Further, the chapter also discusses the diagnostic and management approaches for gallstone diseases, with a focus on the common bile duct involvement. Additionally, we will examine the evolving management strategies for the CBD stones, from traditionally open surgical approaches to minimally invasive laparoscopic and robotic-assisted techniques. By understanding the diagnostic criteria and treatment options available, healthcare providers can make informed decisions to optimize patient care and improve clinical.

2. Etiopathology

2.1 Formation of gallstones

Gallstones are formed when there is an excess of cholesterol in the liver, due to which not all of the cholesterol can be converted into primary, secondary, and tertiary bile acids through hydroxylation. As a result, the excess accumulates and precipitates out of the solution, along with other bile products. These products act as a nucleating factor for the stone formation, in addition to prostaglandins and arachidonyl lecithin, which also serve to promote crystallization [4].

2.1.1 Types of gallstone

While cholesterol is the primary component of gallstones in most cases, there are three major types of gallstones that are typically seen.

- *Cholesterol stones:* typically yellow in color and can be up to 4.5 cm in size. They are primarily composed of cholesterol, along with other components such as calcium salts, bile pigments, and fatty acids [5].

- *Pigment stones:* pigment stones are typically in either brown or black color as they are primarily composed of bilirubin and calcium salts, along with a protein network that holds the structure together. *Black stones* are typically found in patients with hemolysis and in sterile conditions in the gallbladder; however, *brown stones*, which are unpolymerized counterparts of black stones, are typically found in any part of the biliary tract, typically after sepsis and bacterial infections caused by anaerobic bacteria [6].

- *Mixed stones:* typically form when a combination of cholesterol and pigment stones is present in the bile. Mixed gallstones may start as cholesterol stones that are introduced to a septic environment filled with anaerobic bacteria, leading to hydrolysis of the bilirubin conjugates and fatty acids. As a result, these cholesterol stones can accumulate calcium salts, leading to the formation of stones that have the composition of both cholesterol and pigment stones [7].

2.2 Mechanisms of migration

Migration of the gallstones is caused primarily due to the constrictions of the gallbladder, leading to the movement of the stone from the gallbladder to the cystic duct. In cases of smaller gallstones, they may be able to transverse the cystic duct without leading to obstructions; however, most larger gallstones are able to obstruct the cystic duct, leading to cholelithiasis [8]. Further movement of the gallstones can lead to choledocholithiasis, where the gallstones are trapped in the common bile duct.

Migration of gallstones is made easier by hypomobility of the gallbladder, which can lead to stasis of the bile, resulting in more accumulation of gallstones and an increased probability of migration of the accumulated stones. Another factor that helps with the migration of stones is dietary factors. Larger intakes of meals rich in fats can lead to more bile production and increased movement of the gallbladder, which can result in migration of the stones into the biliary ducts [9].

2.3 Primary vs. secondary choledocholithiasis

Primary choledocholithiasis: refers to the situation where the stones are formed directly within the biliary tract, more specifically within the common bile duct. It is typically more common in Asian populations and can be a result of stasis of bile, bacterial infection, or any biliary abnormalities or dysfunctions. Research has found that primary choledocholithiasis is more commonly seen in patients who are older and have increased BMI [2, 10].

Secondary choledocholithiasis: a condition where the primary gallstones formed in the gallbladder later migrate into the common bile duct, resulting in a blockage. Patients with surgical intervention to remove gallstones tend to be more prone to secondary choledocholithiasis. Other factors such as obesity, female sex, pregnancy, and genetic conditions also play a role in increased risk of secondary choledocholithiasis [2].

2.4 Hormonal factors

The incidence of choledocholithiasis tends to be higher in women as opposed to men due to the increased estrogen levels in the body. Increased levels of estrogen in the body, either due to pregnancy or birth control pills, can lead to the accumulation of cholesterol in the bile or can further result in stasis of the gallbladder as well [11].

3. Incidence rate of choledocholithiasis

Choledocholithiasis occurs in 4.6 to 18.8% of patients undergoing cholecystectomy, with its incidence rising in patients with cholelithiasis as they age [12]. Cholelithiasis is more prevalent among females, pregnant individuals, older patients, and those with elevated serum lipid levels. Cholesterol stones are commonly seen in obese patients, those with low physical activity, or individuals who have recently undergone significant weight loss. Black pigment stones are often found in patients with cirrhosis, those receiving total parenteral nutrition, and individuals who have had an ileal resection. Brown pigment primary common bile duct stones are typically associated with bacterial nucleating factors [13, 14].

Globally, approximately 6% of the population is affected by gallstones, with higher rates observed in females and in South America. The incidence of gallstones may be on the rise. A global study by Wang et al. (2023) found that the prevalence of gallstones is 6.1%, higher in females (7.6%) than in males (5.4%), in South America (11.2%) than in Asia (5.1%), in upper-middle-income countries (8.9%) than in high-income countries (4.0%), and increases with age. The incidence was 0.47 per 100 person-years, with an increasing trend in more recent studies [15].

3.1 Global incidence rates

Choledocholithiasis, the presence of gallstones in the common bile duct, is a significant global health concern. While exact global incidence rates are difficult to determine, studies suggest that the condition affects approximately 4.6 to 18.8% of patients undergoing cholecystectomy. The incidence of choledocholithiasis tends to rise with age, and it is more common in females. Geographic variations also influence the incidence, with higher rates observed in regions where cholelithiasis is more prevalent, such as in North America and Europe. Additionally, choledocholithiasis is commonly associated with other factors like obesity, elevated serum lipid levels, and pregnancy.

Between 1990 and 2019, the global burden of gallbladder and biliary tract diseases (GABD), including choledocholithiasis, increased considerably. Incident cases and age-standardized incidence rates (ASIR) rose by 97 and 58.9%, respectively, during this period. Despite a decrease in age-standardized prevalence rates (ASPR) and age-standardized years lived with disability (ASYR), the number of prevalent cases and years lived with disability (YLDs) continued to rise. The highest ASIR for GABD was recorded in Italy, while the United Kingdom had the highest ASPR and ASYR. Furthermore, the burden of the disease was more significant in low-SDI (socio-demographic index) regions, and females experienced a notably higher burden than males [16].

3.2 Risk groups and demographics

The traditional risk factors for gallstone disease are often summarized by the four "F's: female, fat, forty, and fertile." Numerous studies have consistently supported these risk factors, with female gender and obesity being key contributors. Additionally, advanced age and gender are non-modifiable factors, while conditions like a "westernized diet" and physical inactivity can serve as modifiable risks. In particular, obesity, hyperinsulinemia, dyslipidemia, and metabolic syndrome have been shown to predispose individuals to cholesterol gallstones. The relationship between these factors and gallstone formation involves a complex interaction of genetic, environmental, and metabolic conditions [17, 18].

Other risk factors include parity, rapid weight loss, and the use of estrogen replacement therapies or oral contraceptives. Certain populations, such as those with a high prevalence of metabolic syndrome or those receiving total parenteral nutrition, are also at greater risk. Ethnic groups, such as Pima Indians and Mexicans, have been shown to have higher incidences of gallstones, indicating a potential genetic predisposition. As research continues to evolve, understanding the various predisposing factors for gallstones remains crucial for developing targeted prevention strategies [17–20].

4. Diagnosis

Diagnosing gallstone disease, especially that of CBD, is difficult just based on clinical assessment. A comprehensive patient assessment is required, which can be done by obtaining a detailed history and performing a thorough physical examination. This evaluation should include inquiries about various symptoms like pain, nausea, vomiting, fever, and any evidence suggestive of jaundice. Pain should be evaluated by asking about the onset, duration, frequency, and severity of the patient's abdominal pain, along with any history of similar episodes. In this scenario, the pain is described as colicky in nature. As per the Rome criteria, this pain is also described as a steady pain, which is located in the epigastric region and/or right upper quadrant, usually lasting at least 30 min [21]. Pain is usually localized to the right upper quadrant (RUQ) of the abdomen, moderate in intensity, and characterized by an intermittent and recurrent pattern. Patients may often report a history of episodes involving epigastric or RUQ discomfort, sometimes extending to include generalized epigastric pain.

A detailed review of systems is essential to uncover associated symptoms. Patients may report jaundice, which manifests as yellowing of the eyes or skin, accompanied by pruritus, nausea, or vomiting. Jaundice occurs when gallstones obstruct the CBD, leading to the backflow of conjugated bilirubin into the bloodstream. Additional symptoms may include clay-colored stools and tea-colored urine, indicative of biliary obstruction. Importantly, jaundice may present in a cyclical or episodic manner.

In cases of cholangitis, patients may exhibit fever, chills, and possibly altered mental status, collectively referred to as Charcot's triad or Reynolds' pentad when accompanied by hypotension and confusion. Gallstones are implicated in approximately 50% of all pancreatitis cases. Pancreatitis secondary to CBD obstruction typically arises at the level of the Ampulla of Vater. The associated pain is localized to the epigastric and mid-abdominal regions, is continuous in nature—in contrast to the colicky pain seen in choledocholithiasis—and frequently radiates to the back. Nausea and vomiting are also common in pancreatitis. Some patients may experience intermittent pain due to transient obstruction within the CBD caused by floating stones or biliary debris.

During the physical examination, the provider should focus on the patient's general appearance, skin, vital signs, and abdominal findings. RUQ tenderness is a significant clinical finding. Systemic signs such as fever, hypotension, and flushed skin suggest the presence of infection or sepsis. A Courvoisier sign, characterized by a palpable gallbladder, may be noted on examination and is often associated with gallbladder distension due to CBD obstruction. The clinician should also assess for hyperthermia, diaphoresis, jaundice, scleral icterus, tachycardia, hypotension, tachypnea, and specific RUQ abdominal tenderness.

A meticulous approach to history-taking and physical examination is critical in identifying the underlying etiology of the patient's symptoms, particularly when dealing with potential biliary tract or pancreatic pathology. Timely recognition and differentiation of these conditions, such as choledocholithiasis, cholangitis, or pancreatitis, can guide appropriate management strategies and improve patient outcomes. After history and physical examination, it is necessary to evaluate the disease preoperatively through serological investigations. A comprehensive set of laboratory tests are performed to evaluate the patient's condition thoroughly. These tests include a white blood cell count, hemoglobin/hematocrit, platelet count, total bilirubin, direct bilirubin, alkaline phosphatase, aspartate aminotransferase (AST), and alanine aminotransferase (ALT). In patients with cholelithiasis, a total bilirubin level exceeding 3 to 4 mg/dL is strongly suggestive of choledocholithiasis [22]. Additionally, gamma-glutamyl transpeptidase (GGT) levels are typically elevated. Elevated total and direct bilirubin and GGT levels demonstrated the highest sensitivities at 94.7 and 97.9%, respectively [23]. Also, a rise in alkaline phosphatase (ALP) levels is demonstrated in cases of choledocholithiasis. However, the positive predictive value of elevated liver function tests is limited, as these abnormalities can occur in a variety of other conditions. Thus, normal liver function test results are useful for excluding choledocholithiasis. If symptoms resolve and liver function tests show a downward trend, this may indicate that the gallstone has spontaneously passed.

Additionally, a serum lipase test should be performed to evaluate gallstone pancreatitis. An international normalized ratio (INR) and prothrombin time can be ordered to assess intrinsic liver function and coagulation status.

Radiological studies play a critical role in diagnosing biliary disease. The initial imaging modality of choice for suspected biliary pathology, including choledocholithiasis, is a transabdominal ultrasound [24]. This non-invasive test is particularly useful for detecting a dilated common bile duct (CBD), defined as a diameter greater than 6 mm, as well as for identifying stones within the duct. However, the detection of CBD stones via ultrasound can be challenging due to interference caused by gas in the duodenum. Despite this limitation, abdominal ultrasound has a reported accuracy of up to 90% for detecting CBD dilation, though its sensitivity for identifying actual stones ranges between 15 and 40% [22].

If clinical suspicion remains high based on the patient's history, physical examination findings, and laboratory results despite a negative ultrasound, further imaging studies should be pursued. Computed tomography (CT) is frequently utilized as a second-line investigation. While it serves as a valuable second-line imaging modality for diagnosing biliary and related pathological conditions, its diagnostic utility is subject to varying interpretations in the medical literature. CT is generally regarded as a supportive rather than a definitive diagnostic tool [25].

Magnetic resonance cholangiopancreatography (MRCP) is an excellent non-invasive diagnostic tool with a sensitivity of approximately 93% and a specificity of 96% for detecting CBD stones. It is considered superior to a CT scan. MRCP provides detailed visualization of the biliary tree and is particularly useful when ultrasound results are inconclusive. Alternatively, an endoscopic ultrasound (EUS) can be performed, which involves introducing an ultrasound probe into the duodenum under endoscopic guidance. Although more invasive than transabdominal ultrasound or MRCP, EUS is highly sensitive and specific for detecting choledocholithiasis, with reported sensitivity and specificity ranging from 85 to 100% [26]. EUS is more useful for stones smaller than 5 mm as compared to MRCP and has a complication rate between 0.1 and 0.3% [27]. Helical CT and CT cholangiography have been found to provide a greater diagnostic advantage, even specificity comparable to that of MRCP [28, 29]. While MRCP and EUS provide a huge diagnostic advantage, they have some limitations too, primarily with high cost and other reasons like restricted availability in non-tertiary care centers and limited accessibility. The technique is diagnostic but not therapeutic; thus, if stones are identified in the CBD, further interventional procedures are required for treatment. MRCP also has practical challenges, including difficulties in handling severely obese patients, claustrophobia, or the presence of metallic foreign bodies or implanted metallic devices. Furthermore, its diagnostic accuracy can be reduced in cases of small stone diameters (<5 mm) or when peri-pancreatic edema is present, which may complicate the identification of CBDS [30].

Various endoscopic procedures are also performed for diagnostic as well as therapeutic purposes. Mostly these endoscopic procedures are invasive in nature. Endoscopic retrograde cholangiopancreatography (ERCP) is one such procedure that involves cannulating the Ampulla of Vater and subsequently the CBD. By injecting contrast medium under fluoroscopic guidance, filling defects are identified. This technique is frequently the preferred method for evaluating suspected choledocholithiasis and serves as both diagnostic as well as therapeutic. Due to its invasive nature and associated risks, ERCP is recommended primarily for patients with a high probability of choledocholithiasis. When performed by expert operators, it can also serve as an effective treatment. It was historically used for detecting CBD stones, but it is now primarily reserved for therapeutic purposes due to its associated risks, including a 10% risk of post-procedure pancreatitis. ERCP remains highly sensitive but is generally avoided unless intervention is necessary [31]. As compared to EUS and MRCP, the diagnostic accuracy of ERCP is comparatively lower, and it is mostly recommended in patients with a high suspicion of choledocholithiasis [32].

For patients undergoing surgical management, such as laparoscopic or open cholecystectomy, an intraoperative cholangiogram can be performed to assess for choledocholithiasis. This procedure involves inserting a catheter into the cystic duct and injecting contrast material to outline the biliary tree. Radiographic images are then obtained to identify filling defects or obstructions and to confirm the flow of contrast into the duodenum. Additionally, intraoperative ultrasound or laparoscopic ultrasound may be employed to detect choledocholithiasis. However, these techniques are operator-dependent and are not commonly performed by general surgeons due to variability in expertise and equipment availability.

5. Management

5.1 Traditional management

Decades ago, cholelithiasis was treated exclusively with open cholecystectomy, while choledocholithiasis was managed through open CBD exploration (OCBDE), typically performed via duodenotomy and sphincterotomy or bilioenteric anastomosis. Although open surgery is now less widely opted for, recent literature suggests it may have advantages over ERCP for CBD stone clearance, with slightly lower morbidity and mortality rates [33]. Open CBD exploration can be performed using either choledochoenterostomy or sphincterotomy, with the choice depending on the surgeon's experience. Some prefer choledochoenterostomy for CBDs larger than 2 cm to create a wide drainage pathway between the bile duct and intestine.

During sphincterotomy, a 1 cm incision is made in the distal sphincter musculature. A catheter or dilator is passed distally, followed by a Kocher maneuver (mobilization of the duodenum) and duodenotomy at the level of the ampulla. The dilator exposes the ampulla in the surgical field, where it is incised along its anterior-superior border, allowing for the removal of impacted stones.

Choledochoenterostomy is commonly performed as a side-to-side choledochoduodenostomy for patients with a dilated CBD and multiple stones. Long-term success depends on adequate drainage to prevent recurrence of jaundice or cholangitis. The most widely used technique involves a side-to-side hand-sutured anastomosis between the supraduodenal CBD and the duodenum. The Kocher maneuver is performed to expose the distal CBD, followed by a choledochotomy of 2–3 cm along the lateral border of the duodenum. The anastomosis is then created using interrupted absorbable sutures.

One of the major complications of this procedure is sump syndrome, caused by food or debris accumulating in the distal CBD. This condition is typically managed endoscopically via ERCP and sphincterotomy. An alternative approach is choledochojejunostomy with a Roux-en-Y loop, though this technique is popularly performed by experienced surgeons.

5.2 Current management scenario

Management of CBD stones is not standardized, and there is no clear gold standard treatment for choledocholithiasis. Below are various treatment modalities used in the management of bile duct stones (**Table 1**). The recent preferred management strategies for CBD stones include minimally invasive surgery, which can be divided into two options. These include intraoperative management of stones in a single session or two sessions.

The two-session strategy involves performing ERCP preoperatively for clearance of CBD followed by an interval laparoscopic cholecystectomy (LC) for cholelithiasis or LC followed by postoperative ERCP. In contrast to this strategy, single-session management includes LC along with laparoscopic common bile duct exploration (LCBDE) in the same session or LC followed by ERCP in the same sitting, which is also known as the rendezvous technique.

Treatment Modalities	Modalities	Characteristics	Effectiveness	Complications	Technical Issues
Medical	Use of ursodeoxycholic acid, chenodeoxycholic acid, and methyl-tert-butyl-ether that act as brilliant cholesterol solvents.	Dissolving cholesterol gallstones and CBD stones (almost in 85–95% of cases).	50–75%	Few toxic side effects and are toxic to the liver and duodenal mucosa to some extent.	Usually have to be paired up with endoscopic or surgical procedures for better outcomes.
Endoscopic Management	ERCP	Pre- or postoperative ERCP with endoscopic biliary sphincterotomy or surgical bile duct clearance and cholecystectomy.	87–97%	Bleeding, duodenal perforation, cholangitis, pancreatitis, and bile duct injury.	Expertise is required, and large stones may require immediate surgical management.
Laparoscopic Common Bile Duct Exploration (LCBDE)	Laparoscopic retrieval of the stones through the transcystic route or the trans-ductal route.	Stones are either retrieved directly by making an incision in the CBD or by passing a flexible choledochoscope through the cystic duct or CBD.	85–95%	CBD laceration, bleeding, stricture formation, and bile leak.	Surgeon's expertise, availability of advanced equipment, variations in biliary anatomy, and the number and size of CBD stones.
Postoperative Evaluation and Management	Postoperative ERCP	Due to inadequate clearance during LCBDE or retained stones are discovered after an operation.	70–75%	Common complications of ERCP, and if the procedure fails, then laparoscopic or open exploration has to be done.	Various complications of ERCP and highly invasive procedures if secondary ERCP fails.
Open Common Bile Duct Exploration	Choledochoenterostomy or sphincterotomy	Involves creating a large opening between the bile duct and intestine.	95%	Sump Syndrome	Surgeon's experience.
Lithotripsy	EHL, ESWL, or Laser Lithotripsy	Involves fragmenting the bile duct stones into a more manageable form through a shock wave.	64–97%	Damage to the bile duct wall.	Advanced equipment, not cost-effective and requires a high level of expertise.

Table 1.
Available treatment modalities for management of CBD stone and their further evaluation [34].

Preoperative ERCP followed by LC is one of the most commonly utilized approaches for managing cholelithiasis with choledocholithiasis globally. Studies have consistently demonstrated that this two-stage strategy is both safe and effective. However, it has certain limitations contributing to the fact that patients are unnecessarily exposed to potentially risky endoscopic procedures. Advancements in diagnostic modalities such as MRCP and EUS have significantly enhanced the visualization of the biliary tract. These techniques offer high sensitivity and specificity for identifying common bile duct stones preoperatively while being less invasive and not requiring specialized instrumentation. This type of intervention can also lead to residual stones due to incomplete ERCP or migration of new stones during the interval between the two procedures.

Preoperative ERCP has been associated with increased conversion rates from LC to open surgery. Furthermore, this approach typically requires two rounds of anesthesia and hospitalization.

Alternatively, LC followed by postoperative ERCP is occasionally employed but is rarely the first-line treatment for combined cholelithiasis and choledocholithiasis. Postoperative ERCP is mainly reserved for situations where intraoperative exploration of the bile duct is unsuccessful or when bile duct stones are detected during LC but cannot be managed at that time.

One-session procedures are believed to be efficient, safe, convenient, and well-accepted by patients, as the two different pathological conditions are resolved in a single surgery with a single anesthesia. It comprises LCBDE, where CBD is laparoscopically explored. The procedure commenced as a standard laparoscopic cholecystectomy. The gallbladder fundus was retracted toward the right shoulder, while Hartmann's pouch was pulled downward and outward toward the right hip. Calot's triangle was meticulously dissected to achieve the "critical view of safety." (**Figure 2**) The cystic artery was clipped and divided.

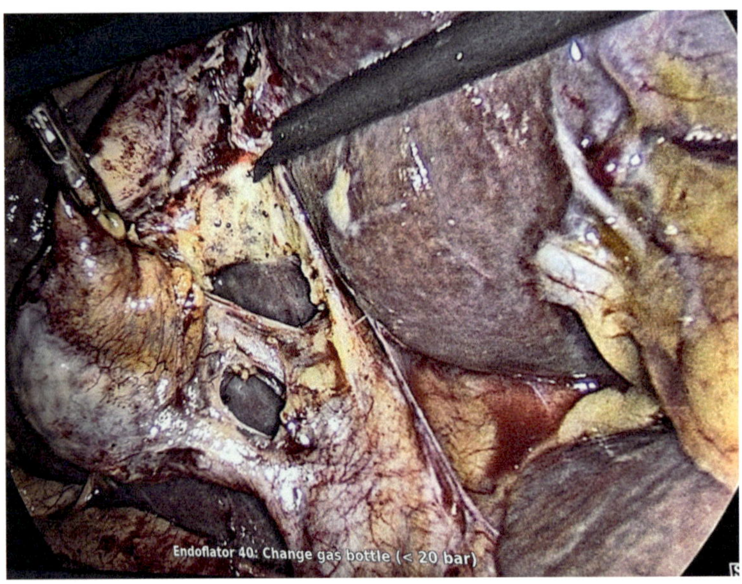

Figure 2.
Critical View of Safety (CVS) Achieved—the cystic artery and cystic duct are clearly visualized connecting to the gallbladder, with the lower one-third of the gallbladder separated from the liver. Clear delineation of Calot's triangle is also evident.

To manage cystic duct stones, the duct was milked toward the gallbladder, ensuring any stones were dislodged. A clip was then applied on the gallbladder side to prevent back slippage of stones into the CBD and to minimize biliary spillage. Digital C-arm fluoroscopy was used to obtain real-time imaging of the biliary tree after contrast injection. The cholangiogram was assessed for filling defects (the "meniscus sign"), as well as the size, location, and number of bile duct stones.

The key point during LCBDE is the longitudinal incision (choledochotomy) that is given on CBD. CBD is supplied at 3 o'clock and 9 o'clock positions by a network of arteries. From above, it is supplied by the right hepatic artery and cystic artery, and from below, the posterior superior pancreaticoduodenal artery, gastroduodenal artery, and retroportal artery. Hence, it is always advised to give a longitudinal incision rather than a transverse incision to avoid bleeding and also the fact that transverse incisions are related more to the development of strictures.

After the entry into the CBD, the stones are milked out through the choledochotomy and retrieved in an endo bag. Further, a choledochoscope can also be inserted to visualize residual stones (**Figure 3**) and can be revived either by milking the duct or through a dormia basket. After the confirmation that the lumen is free of any stones, the choledochotomy is sutured using absorbable sutures. Sometimes a stent or a T-tube endoprosthesis is also placed before the closure into the CBD lumen to prevent any strictures, and the stent is later removed through ERCP.

Many surgeons also prefer a less invasive route, which involves a transcystic introduction of a flexible choledochoscope to visualize the CBD lumen (**Figure 4**). It prevents choledochotomy and further reduces the risks of bile duct injury.

Currently, endoscopic sphincterotomy or endoscopic papillary balloon dilation represents the first-line treatment for initial primary choledocholithiasis, while the LCBDE should be performed for large stones, keeping the sphincter of Oddi intact [35].

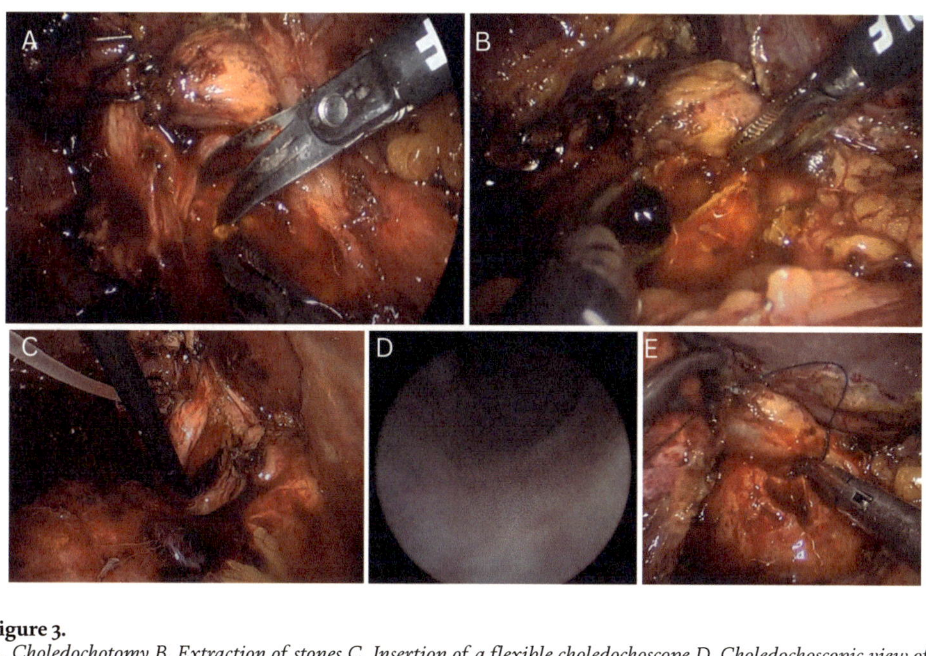

Figure 3.
A. Choledochotomy B. Extraction of stones C. Insertion of a flexible choledochoscope D. Choledochoscopic view of the inside of CBD E. Closing the choledochotomy.

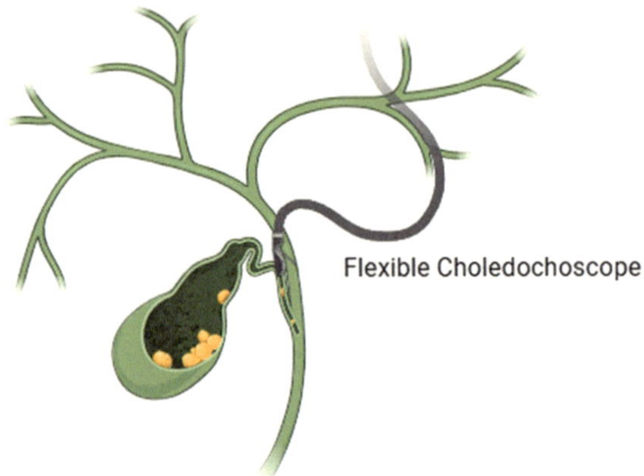

Figure 4.
Illustration of insertion of choledochoscope and retrieval of stone through transcystic approach.

Recent advancements in treatment also include performing ERCP during LC, which is also known as the *rendezvous technique*. This approach requires single hospitalization and single anesthesia, hence making it a safe and effective treatment modality. For this intervention, opening up the duct is not usually required because stones are retrieved by ERCP mainly, and if failed to do so, the bile duct is opened laparoscopically in the same setting, which saves the patient from two different surgical procedures and is cost-effective. Several variations of the rendezvous technique have been developed. In one of the approaches, after advancing the endoscopic sphincterotome over the guidewire through the papilla, an endoscopic sphincterotomy is performed under direct visualization using a simultaneously positioned duodenoscope. Compared to conventional ERCP, the rendezvous technique offers advantages such as improved cannulation in the supine position and a reduced incidence of post-procedural pancreatitis.

Lithotripsy is also considered an ideal management approach for common bile duct stones, as it resolves the condition without disrupting the CBD wall or requiring a sphincterotomy. However, it is not a definitive treatment for cholecysto-choledocholithiasis, as the stone formation is secondary to lithogenic bile in the gallbladder, leading to a high recurrence rate. Additionally, fragmenting gallbladder stones may increase their migration into the bile duct. One key advantage of lithotripsy is that it can often be performed in a single session. While it does not eliminate the need for cholecystectomy, it serves as a valuable alternative for patients who have already undergone the procedure or for whom surgery is not an option. However, its availability is limited by the need for specialized equipment and skilled personnel.

Several techniques are used for stone fragmentation, including mechanical, electrohydraulic, laser, and extracorporeal shock-wave lithotripsy.

- *Endoscopic mechanical lithotripsy* is typically performed when endoscopic sphincterotomy fails. A Dormia basket or balloon catheter is used to capture and fragment stones, achieving bile duct clearance. However, failure can occur with stones larger than 3 cm or those impacted in the CBD [27].

- *Endoscopic electrohydraulic lithotripsy* is an option for difficult cases, using a high-frequency electrohydraulic shock wave probe.

- *Endoscopic laser lithotripsy* is used for large stones under fluoroscopic guidance to minimize heat-induced biliary damage. Recent advances in single-operator steerable cholangioscopy have improved safety by allowing direct visual guidance. Laser lithotripsy is also being explored in laparoscopic, open, and percutaneous procedures.

- *Extracorporeal shock-wave lithotripsy* is employed for difficult stones using ultrasound or fluoroscopic guidance. Modern lithotripters use water-filled compressible bags, but due to patient discomfort, general anesthesia is often required. Contraindications include portal thrombosis and umbilical plexus varices. Potential adverse events include transient biliary colic, subcutaneous bruising, cardiac arrhythmia, self-limited hemobilia, cholangitis, ileus, and pancreatitis. Currently, extracorporeal shock-wave lithotripsy is not considered a first-line treatment for difficult bile duct stones.

5.3 Future is here

With the introduction of robotic-assisted surgery, robotic-assisted cholecystectomy and common bile duct exploration (RC-CBDE) have also been introduced recently. It aims to overcome technical challenges by offering enhanced 3D visualization and articulated instruments, which may improve surgical precision. The benefits of robotic assisted surgery (RAS) include enhanced visualization and improved ergonomics, facilitating precise choledochotomy closure. This may help reduce complications and encourage the broader adoption of common bile duct exploration, a previously underutilized and technically challenging procedure [36].

6. Conclusions

In conclusion, the diagnosis of gallstone disease, particularly involving the CBD, necessitates a comprehensive and systematic approach that combines detailed patient history, clinical examination, laboratory testing, and imaging studies. Recognizing characteristic symptoms such as colicky abdominal pain, jaundice, and signs of pancreatitis or cholangitis is crucial for guiding the evaluation process. Laboratory tests, including liver function tests and serum lipase, along with imaging modalities like transabdominal ultrasound, are integral to confirming the diagnosis and determining the appropriate management strategy. Timely intervention is vital to mitigate complications and improve patient outcomes, underscoring the importance of thorough clinical assessment in suspected biliary pathology.

Acknowledgements

I extend my deepest gratitude to all those who have contributed to the development of this chapter. I am especially grateful to my mentors and colleagues, whose expertise and insights have greatly enriched the content. Their invaluable guidance has shaped my understanding of surgical techniques and principles.

I would also like to acknowledge the dedicated surgical teams and healthcare professionals who work tirelessly to advance patient care. Their commitment to excellence and innovation continues to inspire and drive progress in the field.

Special thanks to the researchers and authors whose work has provided a strong foundation for this chapter. Their contributions to the field of surgery have been instrumental in shaping current knowledge and best practices.

Lastly, I am deeply appreciative of my family and friends for their unwavering support and encouragement throughout this endeavor. Their patience and belief in my work have been a source of constant motivation.

To all who have played a role, directly or indirectly, in the completion of this chapter—thank you.

Conflict of interest

Authors declare that they have no competing interests related to the content of this article. No conflicts of interest, financial ties, or funding sources have influenced the results or interpretations presented in this manuscript.

Author details

Raghav Bansal[1*], Palak Kirti Jain[2], Abhirami Babu[3], Vedant Sachin Kasmalkar[3] and Samridhi Mahajan[1]

1 Department of General Surgery, Adesh Institute of Medical Sciences and Research, Bathinda, Punjab, India

2 Manipal University College Malaysia, Bukit Baru, Melaka, Malaysia

3 Our Lady of Fatima University, College of Medicine, Manila, Philippines

*Address all correspondence to: raghavbansal2001@gmail.com

References

[1] Cleveland Clinic. Choledocholithiasis: Symptoms, Causes & Treatment. Cleveland Clinic (Health Library); Available from: https://my.clevelandclinic.org/health/diseases/24210-choledocholithiasis

[2] Molvar C, Glaenzer B. Choledocholithiasis:Evaluation,treatment, and outcomes. Seminars in Interventional Radiology. 2016;**33**(4):268-276. DOI: 10.1055/s-0036-1592329

[3] McNicoll CF, Pastorino A, Farooq U, Froehlich MJ, St Hill CR. Choledocholithiasis. In: StatPearls [Internet]. Treasure Island (FL): StatPearls Publishing; 2023. Available from: https://www.ncbi.nlm.nih.gov/books/NBK441961/

[4] Jones MW, Weir CB, Ghassemzadeh S. Gallstones (Cholelithiasis). In: StatPearls [Internet]. Treasure Island (FL): StatPearls Publishing; 2024. Available from: https://www.ncbi.nlm.nih.gov/books/NBK459370/

[5] Kumar R, Abbas A. Gallstone ileus: A rare cause of mechanical bowel obstruction. Radiology Case Reports. 2008;**3**(4):256. DOI: 10.1016/j.radcr.2008.08.001

[6] Vitek L, Carey MC. New pathophysiological concepts underlying pathogenesis of pigment gallstones. Clinics and Research in Hepatology and Gastroenterology. 2012;**36**(2):122-129. DOI: 10.1016/j.clinre.2011.08.010

[7] Medscape. Choledocholithiasis. Available from: https://emedicine.medscape.com/article/175667-overview

[8] Taylor TV, Armstrong CP. Migration of gall stones. British Medical Journal (Clinical Research Ed.). 1987;**294**(6583):1320-1322. DOI: 10.1136/bmj.294.6583.1320

[9] MSD Manual. Cholelithiasis. In: MSD Manual Professional Version. Rahway, NJ, USA: MSD Manual; 2023. Available from: https://www.msdmanuals.com/professional/hepatic-and-biliary-disorders/gallbladder-and-bile-duct-disorders/cholelithiasis#Symptoms-and-Signs_v901781

[10] Ruiz Pardo J, García Marín A, Ruescas García FJ, et al. Differences between residual and primary choledocholithiasis in cholecystectomy patients. Revista Española de Enfermedades Digestivas. 2020;**112**(8):615-619. DOI: 10.17235/reed.2020.6760/2019

[11] Johns Hopkins Medicine. Gallstones. Available from: https://www.hopkinsmedicine.org/health/conditions-and-diseases/gallstones

[12] McNicoll CF, Pastorino A, Farooq U, et al. Choledocholithiasis. In: StatPearls [Internet]. Treasure Island (FL): StatPearls Publishing; 2025. Available from: https://www.ncbi.nlm.nih.gov/books/NBK441961/ [Accessed: July 10, 2023]

[13] van Dijk AH, de Reuver PR, Besselink MG, van Laarhoven KJ, Harrison EM, Wigmore SJ, et al. Assessment of available evidence in the management of gallbladder and bile duct stones: A systematic review of international guidelines. HPB: The Official Journal of the International Hepato Pancreato Biliary Association. 2017;**19**(4):297-309

[14] Jinfeng Z, Yin Y, Chi Z, Junye G. Management of impacted common

bile duct stones during a laparoscopic procedure: A retrospective cohort study of 377 consecutive patients. International Journal of Surgery. 2016;**32**:1-5

[15] Wang X et al. Global epidemiology of gallstones in the 21st century: A systematic review and meta-analysis. Clinical Gastroenterology and Hepatology. 2024;**22**(8):1586-1595

[16] Li ZZ, Guan LJ, Ouyang R, Chen ZX, Ouyang GQ, Jiang HX. Global, regional, and national burden of gallbladder and biliary diseases from 1990 to 2019. World Journal of Gastrointestinal Surgery. 2023;**15**(11):2564-2578. DOI: 10.4240/wjgs.v15.i11.2564

[17] Sherlock S. Diseases of the Liver and Biliary System. 3rd ed. Oxford: Blackwell Scientific Publications; 1963

[18] Pak M, Lindseth G. Risk factors for Cholelithiasis. Gastroenterology Nursing. 2016;**39**(4):297-309. DOI: 10.1097/SGA.0000000000000235

[19] Volzke H, Baumeister SE, Alte D, Hoffmann W, Schwahn C, Simon P, et al. Independent risk factors for gallstone formation in a region with high cholelithiasis prevalence. Digestion. 2005;**71**(2):97-105

[20] Di Ciaula A, Wang DQH, Wang HH, Leonilde B, Portincasa P. Targets for current pharmacological therapy in cholesterol gallstone disease. Gastroenterology Clinics of North America. 2010;**39**(2):245-264. DOI: 10.1016/j.gtc2010.02.005

[21] Rome Group for Epidemiology and Prevention of Cholelithiasis (GREPCO). The epidemiology of gallstone disease in Rome, Italy. Part II. Factors associated with the disease. Hepatology. 1988;**8**(4):907-913

[22] Park CH. The management of common bile duct stones. The Korean Journal of Gastroenterology. 2018;**71**(5):260-263. DOI: 10.4166/kjg.2018.71.5.260

[23] Yang MH, Chen TH, Wang SE, Tsai YF, Su CH, Wu CW, et al. Biochemical predictors for absence of common bile duct stones in patients undergoing laparoscopic cholecystectomy. Surgical Endoscopy. 2008;**22**:1620-1624

[24] Maple JT, Ben-Menachem T, Anderson MA, Appalaneni V, Banerjee S, Cash BD, et al. The role of endoscopy in the evaluation of suspected choledocholithiasis. Gastrointestinal Endoscopy. 2010;**71**(1):1-9

[25] Mitchell SE, Clark RA. A comparison of computed tomography and sonography in choledocholithiasis. American Journal of Roentgenology. 1984;**142**(4):729-733

[26] Lammert F, Gurusamy K, Ko CW, Miquel JF, Méndez-Sánchez N, Portincasa P, et al. Gallstones. Nature Reviews Disease Primers. 2016;**2**(1):1-7

[27] Masuda S, Koizumi K, Shionoya K, Jinushi R, Makazu M, Nishino T, et al. Comprehensive review on small common bile duct stones. World Journal of Gastroenterology. 2023;**29**(13):1955-1968. DOI: 10.3748/wjg.v29.i13.1955

[28] Kondo S, Isayama H, Akahane M, Toda N, Sasahira N, Nakai Y, et al. Detection of common bile duct stones: Comparison between endoscopic ultrasonography, magnetic resonance cholangiography, and helical-computed-tomographic cholangiography. European Journal of Radiology. 2005;**54**(2):271-275

[29] Yamamoto N, Hirano K, Komatsu Y, Tada M, Yoshida H. Detection

of common bile duct stones: Comparison between endoscopic ultrasonography, magnetic resonance cholangiography, and helical-computed-tomographic cholangiography. European Journal of Radiology. 2005;**54**(2):271-275

[30] Polistina FA, Frego M, Bisello M, Manzi E, Vardanega A, Perin B. Accuracy of magnetic resonance cholangiography compared to operative endoscopy in detecting biliary stones, a single center experience and review of literature. World Journal of Radiology. 2015;7(4):70

[31] Williams EJ, Taylor S, Fairclough P, Hamlyn A, Logan RF, Martin D, et al. Risk factors for complication following ERCP; results of a large-scale, prospective multicenter study. Endoscopy. 2007;**39**(09):793-801

[32] Karakan T, Cindoruk M, Alagozlu H, Ergun M, Dumlu S, Unal S. EUS versus endoscopic retrograde cholangiography for patients with intermediate probability of bile duct stones: A prospective randomized trial. Gastrointestinal Endoscopy. 2009;**69**(2):244-252

[33] Dasari BVM, Tan CJ, Gurusamy KS, Martin DJ, Kirk G, McKie L, et al. Surgical versus endoscopic treatment of bile duct stones. Cochrane Database of Systematic Reviews. 2013;(12):Art. No.: CD003327. DOI: 10.1002/14651858.CD003327.pub4 [Accessed 03 May 2025]

[34] Shojaiefard A, Esmaeilzadeh M, Ghafouri A, Mehrabi A. Various techniques for the surgical treatment of common bile duct stones: A meta review. Gastroenterology Research and Practice. 2009;**2009**:1-12. DOI: 10.1155/2009/840208

[35] Cianci P, Restini E. Management of cholelithiasis with choledocholithiasis: Endoscopic and surgical approaches. World Journal of Gastroenterology. 2021;**27**(28):4536-4554. DOI: 10.3748/wjg.v27.i28.4536

[36] Lewis H, Latif J, Bandlamudi N, Bhatti I, Awan A. 407 robotic assisted cholecystectomy and common bile duct exploration for single stage Management of Complex Gallstone Disease. British Journal of Surgery. 2023;**110**(7):znad258.451. DOI: 10.1093/bjs/znad258.451

Chapter 7

Total Pancreatectomy for Chronic Pancreatitis: Surgical Technique and Recent Advances

Aamir Khan

Abstract

Total pancreatectomy (TP) is an important surgical intervention for refractory chronic pancreatitis (CP), offering durable pain relief despite the inevitable metabolic consequences of pancreatic insufficiency and potentially post-pancreatectomy diabetes. This chapter describes the evolution of TP for chronic pancreatitis, emphasizing the paradigm-shifting integration of islet autotransplantation (TPIAT), which preserves endocrine function in a vast number of patients. Modern indications focus on patients with intractable pain, diffuse calcifications, or genetic CP variants unresponsive to medical or endoscopic interventions. The chapter systematically details distinct role of TP in chronic pancreatitis including preoperative optimization, surgical techniques with distinctions between standard TP and TPIAT-specific vascular preservation. Key steps and differences in vascular dissection to bowel reconstruction are outlined, alongside emerging minimally invasive (laparoscopic/robotic) approaches. Postoperative management highlights glycemic control, enzyme replacement, and novel anti-inflammatory therapies (e.g., Anakinra) to enhance islet survival. Outcomes data demonstrate excellent improvement in quality of life and pain reduction, endocrine preservation with IAT, and excellent long term survival. Total pancreatectomy remains a very important and viable treatment option for patients suffering from refractory chronic or recurrent acute pancreatitis.

Keywords: total pancreatectomy, chronic pancreatitis, islet cell transplant, exocrine pancreatic insufficiency, robotic-assisted

1. Introduction

Chronic pancreatitis (CP) represents a complex, progressive inflammatory disorder of the pancreas marked by irreversible fibrotic replacement of functional parenchyma, ultimately leading to exocrine and endocrine insufficiency [1]. The disease manifests most prominently through debilitating abdominal pain - often refractory to conventional therapies - which significantly diminishes patients' quality of life while predisposing to severe complications including pancreatic duct strictures, pseudocyst formation, biliary obstruction, and malignant transformation [2, 3]. Contemporary management requires a multidisciplinary paradigm encompassing medical therapy, endoscopic intervention, and surgical strategies tailored to disease severity and anatomical involvement [3].

The etiology of CP follows a multifactorial model where alcohol consumption accounts for 60–70% of cases in Western populations, though emerging evidence highlights critical interactions between environmental triggers and genetic susceptibility [4]. Hereditary forms, representing 10–15% of cases, frequently involve mutations in cationic trypsinogen (PRSS1), serine protease inhibitor Kazal-type 1 (SPINK1), cystic fibrosis transmembrane conductance regulator (CFTR), and chymotrypsin C (CTRC) genes, which disrupt pancreatic autoprotection mechanisms against premature enzyme activation [5, 6]. Obstructive etiologies (e.g., pancreatic duct strictures, sphincter of Oddi dysfunction) and metabolic disorders (notably hypertriglyceridemia and hypercalcemia) constitute other well-characterized pathways [7]. The necrosis-fibrosis hypothesis posits that recurrent acute pancreatitis episodes initiate a self-perpetuating cycle of inflammation, acinar cell loss, and fibrotic replacement - a process amplified by oxidative stress and cytokine-mediated signaling [8, 9]. Tropical pancreatitis, endemic to equatorial regions, presents distinct epidemiological patterns potentially linked to cassava toxicity, micronutrient deficiencies, and genetic polymorphisms [10]. Despite diagnostic advances, approximately 20–30% of cases remain classified as idiopathic, though many likely represent undetected genetic variants or atypical autoimmune mechanisms [11].

The surgical approach to CP has undergone remarkable transformation since the first successful total pancreatectomy (TP) by Rockey in 1943 for malignancy - a procedure initially burdened by 25–40% mortality due to technical challenges and inadequate metabolic support [12, 13]. The development of purified insulin and enteric-coated pancreatic enzymes in the 1970s–1980s enabled broader application for benign disease, while Puestow's longitudinal pancreaticojejunostomy (1958) and Beger's duodenum-preserving pancreatic head resection (1980) established organ-sparing alternatives [14, 15]. A revolutionary advance came with Sutherland's 1977 demonstration of islet autotransplantation (TPIAT), which sought to mitigate the inevitable type3c diabetes following TP by reinfusing a patient's own isolated islets [16]. The twenty-first century has witnessed paradigm shifts through minimally invasive approaches (laparoscopic/robotic TP), enhanced recovery protocols, and sophisticated glucose monitoring systems that collectively reduced mortality to <5% at high-volume centers [17, 18]. These innovations have refined TP's role in CP management, particularly for diffuse small-duct disease or genetic forms where parenchymal preservation proves unfeasible [19].

Modern indications for TP in CP prioritize patients with intractable pain refractory to multimodal analgesia and endoscopic therapy, particularly when imaging demonstrates diffuse calcifications or ductal abnormalities precluding limited resections [20]. The procedure's metabolic consequences - including brittle diabetes and pancreatic exocrine insufficiency - remain substantial but increasingly manageable through closed-loop insulin systems, continuous glucose monitoring, and microencapsulated enzyme formulations [21]. TPIAT has emerged as a transformative strategy, with 30–40% of recipients achieving insulin independence when >5000 islet equivalents/kg are transplanted, while >80% experience significant pain reduction [22, 23]. Ongoing research explores nerve-targeted interventions alternative islet implantation sites, and regenerative approaches that may further optimize outcomes [21, 24].

This chapter systematically examines the technical execution, perioperative considerations, and evolving innovations that define TP's role in chronic pancreatitis.

2. Preoperative planning

Involvement of a multidisciplinary team is extremely important for optimal outcome of this operation. Patients should be evaluated for any major prohibitive cardiopulmonary comorbidities and evaluated accordingly. Patients should be vaccinated against encapsulated bacteria (*Streptococcus pneumoniae*, *Neisseria meningitidis* and Hemophilus influenzae type B,) to prevent risk of overwhelming post splenectomy sepsis, if splenectomy is needed or planned [25]. These should be given at least 2 weeks before surgery. Assessment of islet function with C-peptide measurements and/or mixed meal tolerance tests is helpful for patients for TPIAT. We offer TPIAT only to patients who have preserved islet function. Abdominal cross sectional imaging with either MRI or CT scan is paramount for surgical planning [26, 27]. For patients with chronic pancreatitis who are planned for autoislet cell transplant, endoscopic ultrasound is also used frequently by many centers to rule out any pancreatic malignancy and assess pancreas tissue [28]. Sometimes, patients are severely malnourished and a period of nutritional prehabilitation is useful to help improve outcomes and post surgical healing and recovery.

3. Surgical technique

The patient is positioned supine with arms either tucked at the side or abducted at less than 90 degrees. After administration of general anesthesia, central venous access, arterial line and Foley catheter is placed. Preoperative antibiotics are given. At author's program, Ampicillin-sulbactam and fluconazole are preferably used.

An upper midline or bilateral subcostal incision is used to gain access to the upper abdomen. A thorough exploration of the peritoneal cavity is performed. Retraction is achieved using one of the self-retaining retractor systems like Thompson or Omnitract retractors.

Total pancreatectomy techniques for chronic pancreatitis differ if islet auto-transplant is being planned as the vascular supply needs to be preserved till the very end to preserve the viability of islets [29].

After good exposure has been set up, we begin our dissection with cholecystectomy. This is achieved by either fundus-first technique or the duct-first technique, as per the surgeon's preference. The cystic duct and artery are ligated and divided separately. Gall bladder is mobilized from the liver bed and removed. Afterwards, initial dissection is focused towards establishing resectability.

The peritoneum over the hepatoduodenal ligament is scored with an electrocautery. The bile duct is circumferentially dissected distally close to pancreas head and encircled with vessel loops. Gastroduodenal artery (GDA) is identified and looped. The right gastric artery is often ligated and divided to aid in exposure of common hepatic artery (CHA). It is important to understand that due to the inflammation from acute or chronic pancreatitis, often the natural tissue plane between these vessels and the pancreas head are obliterated and extreme care should be taken in handling these vessels and structures. Once the GDA and the CHA are dissected free, the portal vein should be visible. The plane between the portal vein and the pancreas neck is explored superiorly as much as it can be done safely. Care should be taken to avoid dissecting too far down superiorly as any bleeding from the portal vein or its tributaries could be difficult to manage at this stage. The proximal splenic artery is similarly dissected and looped around.

Hepatic flexure of the colon is mobilized and a full Kocker maneuver is performed to mobilize the duodenum and the pancreas head from its retroperitoneal attachment (**Figure 1a**). This allows a good assessment of the pancreas head for any masses or lesions. Kocherization maneuver is continued medially until the proximal left renal vein is exposed anteriorly. In the present era of advanced pancreatic imaging, this is not as important for pancreatitis surgery as it is for pancreas cancer surgery but still relevant not only to assess the inflammation/resectability but also gives a potential way of bleeding control by putting pressure on the pancreas head/neck if there is any such difficult to control bleeding from pancreatic portal tributaries while trying to create the tunnel between portal vein and pancreas neck (**Figure 1b**).

Next, lesser sac is entered by exposing the plane between the stomach and the colon. This can sometimes be completely obliterated because of prior pancreatitis or pseudocyst or cystgastrostomies. Careful dissection is done to re-establish this plane in difficult cases with attention to avoid creating any unnecessary mesenteric windows or pancreatic capsular tears. The gastrocolic ligament is divided along the gastroepiploic vein which is different from cancer operations where the omentum is divided off from the transverse colon. We prefer to use LigaSure to divide this as it contains small venous tributaries from the epiploic vessels. Dissection is carried out until the short gastric vessels are reached and they are divided closer to the spleen using the LigaSure device. At this time the greater curvature of the stomach is freed completely. Dissection is carried along the left epiploic vein until it reaches the superior mesenteric vein (SMV). Sometimes, the epiploic vein first joins the middle colic vein to form a common trunk that drains into the SMV. Following this plane allows a safe exposure of the SMV and inferior border of the pancreas.

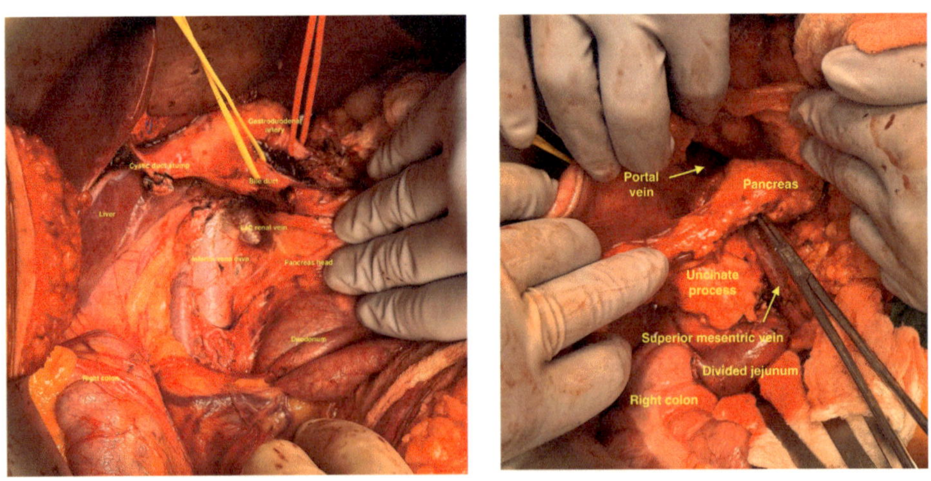

(a) (b)

Figure 1.
(a): Head of pancreas and duodenum mobilized medially exposing inferior vena cava and left renal vein, along with dissected out bile duct and gastroduodenal artery. (b): Creating dissection plane between portal vein and the pancreas neck.

DOI: http://dx.doi.org/10.5772/intechopen.1011017

Dissection is carried carefully along the anterior surface of the SMV and portal vein to establish the tunnel posterior to the neck of the pancreas. An umbilical tape or a Penrose drain can be passed around to establish a sling maneuver [30]. This establishes resectability and further dissection or division of structures depends upon whether islet cell auto-transplant is planned or not. If islet cell auto-transplant is considered then the vessels (GDA, splenic vein and artery) need to be left intact until before the removal of the organ. Without islet cell transplant however, the vessels can be divided to ease further dissection.

Ligament of Trietz is identified and a GIA stapler is used to divide the proximal jejunum about 10 cm distally. The divided proximal jejunal stump is freed from its mesentery and the ligament of Trietz and then passed medially posterior to the mesenteric vessels. Next the stomach antrum is divided using a GIA stapler.

Pylorus preservation is subject to surgeon or program preference, as well as any prior gastric procedures likes feeding gastrostomies or cystgastrostomies. We do not routinely perform pylorus preservation, since quite a number of patients tend to have gastroparesis and performing an antrectomy not only helps with that but also helps to have better efficacy of pancreatic enzymes since removing antrum also gets rid of the most acid producing cells of the stomach.

The pancreas head and uncinate process are reflected medially and the SMV is separated from the uncinate process. As this surgery is not done for cancer, lymph node dissection is not needed. Our preference is to use suture ligatures to divide this tissue but any energy device like Harmonic Scalpel or LigaSure can also be used. Dissection is carried cephalad along the plane of pancreatic tissue merging with perivascular lymphatic tissue of SMA. Inferior pancreaticoduodenal vessels will be encountered and will usually need additional clips or suture ligature. Common bile duct is divided and this further facilitates the lateral retraction of the pancreas head to expose the plane between portal vein and the pancreas head. Surgeon should be mindful of any aberrant or replaced right hepatic artery coming off the SMA that will need to be preserved. I find it useful to keep SMA pushed medially with the tip of fingers while the rest of the left hand is retracting the pancreas head. Once all of the pancreas head is mobilized, attention is turned towards mobilization of the pancreas tail and body. The inferior border of the pancreas body/tail is mobilized by dissecting it free from its retroperitoneal tissue attachments. The inferior mesenteric vein is usually encountered during this dissection and preferably preserved, unless it is joining splenic vein too far distally in which case it can be ligated. Once the dissection reaches the splenic flexure, colon is freed from spleen by dividing the spleno-colic tissue. Next spleen is mobilized by holding it with the left hand and pulled medially to expose the retroperitoneal plane behind it (**Figure 2**). The tissue is scored with electrocautery and it usually exposes the avascular plane behind the pancreas. The splenic vein is encircled just distal to the point of attachment with the inferior mesenteric vein or roughly at the point where there is still 2–3 cms of splenic vein stump left.

At this time pancreas is ready to come out and is only attached with GDA, splenic artery and splenic vein. The GDA, splenic artery and splenic vein are ligated in that order and the pancreas is removed (**Figure 3**). Next the organ handed over to the islet isolation team for flushing, preparation and packaging for islet auto-transplant later. The isolation procedure is done as per the standard method described by Riccordi [31]. A detailed description of that is beyond the scope of this chapter.

Next attention is turned towards reconstruction to re-establish gastrointestinal continuity. Our preference is to do reconstruction in a Roux-en-Y configuration. This is achieved by using the previously stapled jejunum and bringing it in a retrocolic

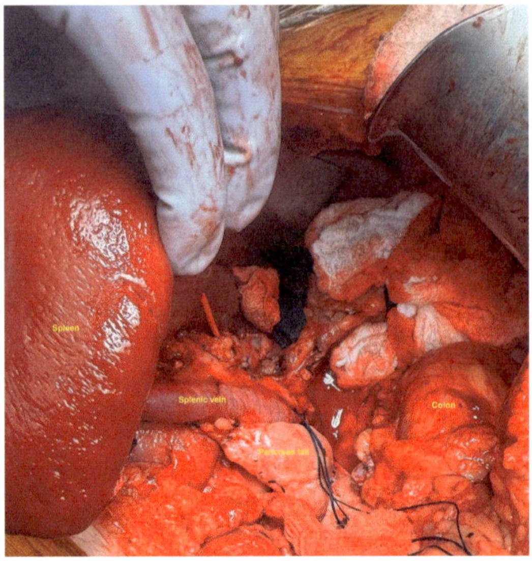

Figure 2.
Spleen and pancreas tail mobilized medially and splenic vessels encircled.

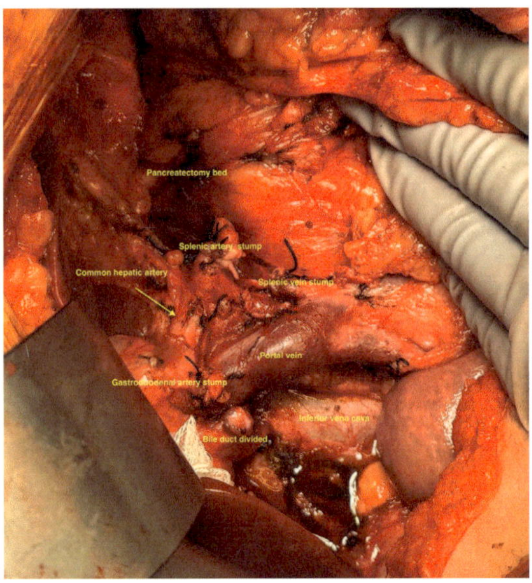

Figure 3.
Pancreas removed and the pancreatectomy bed.

fashion through an opening in the mesocolon to create a gastrojejunostomy. This is performed in two layers in an end-to side fashion using absorbable 4-0 PDS suture for the inner full thickness layer and interrupted 3-0 silk sutures for the outer seromuscular layer (**Figure 4a, b**). A Roux limb is created by dividing the jejunum about 45 cms distal from the gastrojejunostomy anastomosis. The distal end is brought through another defect created in the mesocolon and a hepaticojeunostomy or choledochojejunostomy is created in an end-to-side fashion (**Figure 5**). Our preferred technique is to use interrupted sutures of 5-0 monofilament sutures either Prolene or PDS.

DOI: http://dx.doi.org/10.5772/intechopen.1011017

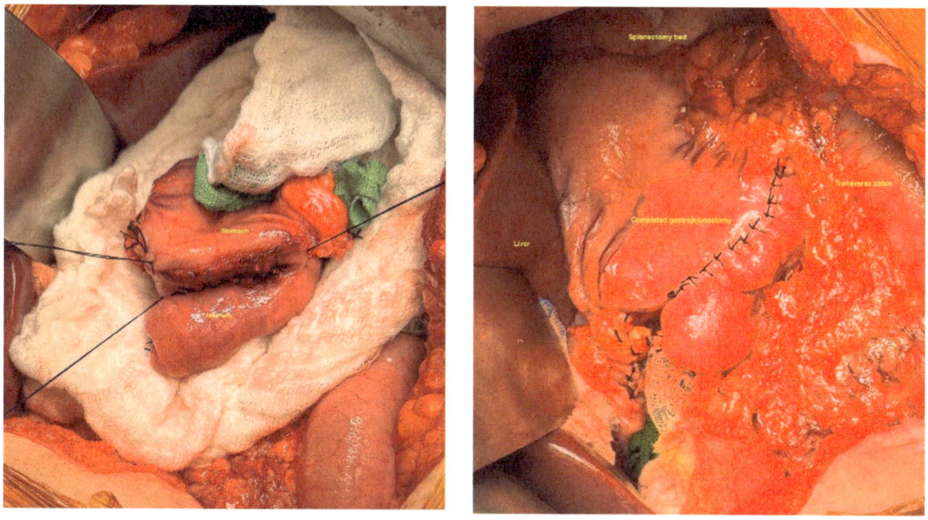

(a) (b)

Figure 4.
(a): Hand sewn gastrojejunostomy started with posterior layer of seromuscular sutures. (b): A two layered hand-sewn gastrojejunostomy completed showing anterior row of seromuscular suture line.

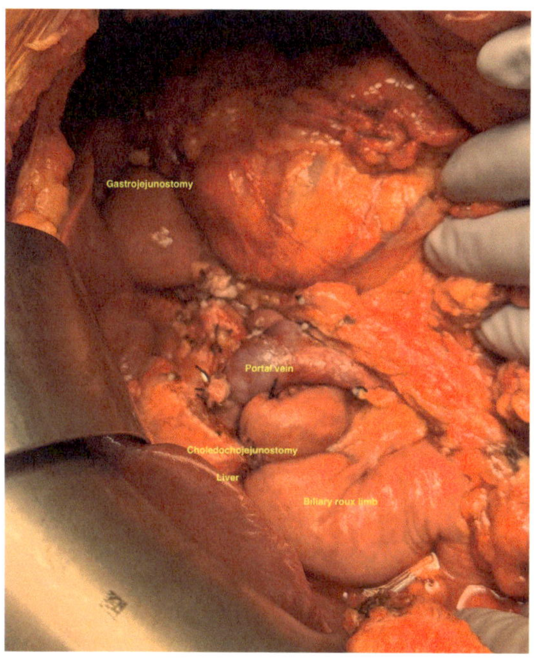

Figure 5.
Completed Roux-en-Y choledochojeunostomy.

Next about 45 cm distal to the bilioenteric anastomosis a side-to-side jejunojejunostomy is created in a two layer fashion with inner full thickness layer with 4-0 PDS suture and outer seromuscular sutures using interrupted 3-0 silk sutures. Both the gastric limb and the biliary limb of the Roux-en-Y reconstruction need to be secured to the mesocolon with a few interrupted non-absorable sutures. Similarly, the mesenteric defect from the jejunojejunostomy as well as the previous ligament of Treitz defect also needs to be closed with a few interrupted silk sutures. At our program we do not generally place any drains. However, drains can be placed at surgeon's discretion if needed.

4. Total pancreatectomy with islet auto-transplant

If islet auto-transplant is being planned, then islets once isolated and ready are infused in the patient's liver through the portal vein. A 6-0 Prolene stay suture is placed on the splenic vein stump or any vein branch draining into the portal venous system. A small angiocatheter usually 14–16 french angiocatheter is placed in the vein and secured using the stay suture. Portal vein pressure is measured at baseline and every 5 minute intervals. If the portal vein pressure goes above 20–25 mmHg, infusion is paused and resumed after an interval. If the portal pressure has not dropped, then alternative sites are used which mostly is either omentum or peritoneum [32]. Once the infusion is finished the catheter is pulled out and the venotomy site is closed using a 6-0 prolene suture.

5. Minimally invasive total pancreatectomy

As experience with minimally invasive pancreatic resections is growing, total pancreatectomy has been also performed using both laparoscopic and robotic approaches. Several reports and case series exist now describing these approaches even for TPIATs as feasible and safe [33]. However, these approaches require a learning curve and should be reserved for surgeons highly experienced in laparoscopy or robotic surgery. The introduction of robotic surgery has addressed many limitations of laparoscopic surgery like avoiding tremors, enhanced 3-dimesional visualization, greater dexterity and ease of suturing, and improved ergonomics and is therefore gaining significant popularity.

Early outcomes, safety and feasibility of the minimally invasive procedures seems comparable to the open procedures. Long term data with larger case numbers is needed to further establish the role of minimally invasive total pancreatectomy with islet cell auto transplant [34–37]. The principals of the surgery remain essentially the same but use of energy devices like Vessel sealer, Harmonic scalpel is much more common for dissection of the uncinate process. Our recommendation is to at least identify inferior pancreaticoduodenal artery and to clip or ligate it separately. Similarly, the vein of belcher or the posterior superior pancreaticoduodenal vein should also be ligated or clipped separately especially for TPIAT since increased portal pressure can cause troublesome bleeding during islet infusion.

6. Postoperative management

Patients need to be monitored very closely for bleeding and for hypoglycemia. Therefore, patients generally are sent to intensive care unit for close monitoring. Patient's glucose levels are monitored hourly and a continuous insulin drip is started.

When islet cell autotransplantation is done, tight glycemic control is especially more important as hyperglycemia can have deleterious effect on islet cells [38]. Diet is slowly advanced starting at clear liquids until a regular diabetic diet is achieved. Once blood glucose levels are stabilized less frequent glucose checks are performed and patients are transitioned to intermittent insulin dosing, if needed. Pain control is more important for this patient population as most of them will be undergoing this surgery for pain control and might have been already on a lot of opioids before. Their management can be tricky and usually requires multimodal analgesia. Consultation with pain management specialists is very helpful. Heparin DVT prophylaxis is started as soon as bleeding risk is minimal. Pancreatic enzyme replacement therapy is started once patient is on a diet. Dose is titrated based on the fat content of the food as well as the resolution of symptoms of steatorrhea. Most formulations of enzymes are available as delayed release formulations and do not always need acid suppressive therapy, but if the steatorrhea and malabsorption continues, it might be worthwhile adding an H2 blocker or proton pump inhibitor also. Antibiotics are given as per the institutional guidelines.

In case an autotransplant is performed, patients are usually also placed on heparin infusion to prevent portal vein thrombosis. A vascular ultrasound is done on postoperative day 1 at our program to assess the patency of the portal vein. Patients also receive Anakinra and etanercept to reduce inflammation and improve islet survival [39].

7. Results and outcomes

Total pancreatectomy mitigates the significant complications of partial pancreatectomies like pancreatic leaks and fistulas, it is still a major procedure with potential for significant morbidity and even mortality. Quality of life after total pancreatectomy has traditionally been perceived to be poor secondary to brittle insulin dependent diabetes and pancreatic insufficiency. However, with advent of islet cell autotransplant, the risk of brittle diabetes can be significantly mitigated. Management of exocrine pancreatic insufficiency has improved also dramatically with advent of good pancreatic enzyme formulations and with our better understanding of their pharmacology.

Several series have reported favorable outcomes for total pancreatectomy with islet autotransplantation for chronic pancreatitis. Improvement in quality of life, reduction in opioid requirements, and pain have been shown by a number of studies. TPIAT has been able to especially avoid the difficulty of managing brittle diabetes associated with apancreatic state. Chinakotla et al. in a series 484 patients reported over 90% pain relief, more than 65% had partial or full betacell function, and significant quality of life improvement [40]. Morgan et al. reported in a cohort of 195 patients of chronic pancreatitis a 5 year survival of 92.3% and a quality of life significantly improved from baseline [41]. Chinakotla also reported in an favorable outcomes in pediatric population in a series of 75 children who underwent TPIAT with over 90% patients reporting improvement in pain and sustained relief from narcotics. About 41.3% achieved insulin independence in that series [22]. Wilson reported no perioperative mortality in a cohort of 166 patients and 94.6% 5 year patient survival [42]. **Table 1** highlights the long term outcomes as described by some major patient series performing total pancreatectomy procedures.

Author	Year	Number of patients	Insulin independence	Narcotic use	5 year survival (%)
Sutherland et al. [43]	2012	409	30% insulin independent at 3 years. 33% partial function	85% improvement in pain. 59% narcotic free at 2 years	90%
Chinakotla et al. [40]	2014	484	¼ patients insulin independent at 10 years but almost 50% had partial islet function	80% narcotic free	90.27%
Wilson et al. [42]	2014	166	38% insulin independent and 38% with partial graft function at 1 year	79% narcotic independent at 5 years	94.6%
Morgan et al. [41]	2018	195	29% at 1 year and 23% at 5 years insulin independent.	Narcotic use significantly decreased.	92.3%
Coluzzi et al. [44]	2023	178	29% insulin independent at 3 years	Daily morphine requirements and pain scores significantly decreased at 3 years.	
Garcia et al. [20]	2013	60	21.6%	45%	Greater than 90%
Sutton et al. [45]	2010	118	25% insulin independent and 44% had partial islet function at almost 2 years	81% experienced little to no pain and 63% were completely narcotic free	1 patient died after 2 years

Table 1.
Long term outcomes after total pancreatectomy with islet autotransplant.

8. Conclusions

Total pancreatectomy (TP) remains a definitive treatment for refractory chronic pancreatitis in adult and pediatric patients, offering durable pain relief in a vast majority of patients despite the inevitable consequences of exocrine insufficiency and diabetes in some patients. The combination with islet autotransplantation (IAT), has improved outcomes by reducing surgical morbidity and preserving endocrine function. The evolution of minimally invasive techniques, particularly robotic surgery has opened a new and an exciting chapter in pancreatic surgery. Ongoing research in islet isolation techniques, preventing damage from innate immunity and inflammation, alternative sites for islet transplant are likely going to further improve the outcomes of this procedure. Although TP is a radical intervention, careful patient selection and ongoing advancements in surgical and metabolic support continue to solidify its role in managing end-stage chronic pancreatitis, balancing the trade-off between pain relief and lifelong metabolic management.

Author details

Aamir Khan
Department of Surgery, Virginia Commonwealth University, Richmond, VA, USA

*Address all correspondence to: aamir.khan@vcuhealth.org

References

[1] Kleeff J, Whitcomb DC, Shimosegawa T, Esposito I, Lerch MM, Gress TM, et al. Chronic pancreatitis. Nature Reviews. Disease Primers. 2017;**3**:17060. DOI: 10.1038/nrdp.2017.60

[2] Drewes AM, Bouwense SAW, Campbell CM, Ceyhan GO, Delhaye M, Demir IE, et al. Guidelines for the understanding and management of pain in chronic pancreatitis. Pancreatology. 2017;**17**(5):720-731. DOI: 10.1016/j.pan.2017.07.006

[3] Hart PA, Conwell DL. Chronic pancreatitis: Managing a difficult disease. The American Journal of Gastroenterology. 2020;**115**(1):49-55. DOI: 10.14309/ajg.0000000000000421

[4] Yadav D, Lowenfels AB. The epidemiology of pancreatitis and pancreatic cancer. Gastroenterology. 2013;**144**(6):1252-1261. DOI: 10.1053/j.gastro.2013.01.068

[5] Whitcomb DC. Genetic risk factors for pancreatic disorders. Gastroenterology. 2013;**144**(6):1292-1302. DOI: 10.1053/j.gastro.2013.01.069

[6] LaRusch J, Lozano-Leon A, Stello K, Moore A, Muddana V, O'Connell M, et al. The common chymotrypsinogen C (CTRC) variant G60G (c.180T) increases risk of chronic pancreatitis but not recurrent acute pancreatitis in a north American population. Clinical and Translational Gastroenterology. 2018;**6**(1):e68. DOI: 10.1038/ctg.2014.13

[7] Forsmark CE. Management of chronic pancreatitis. Gastroenterology. 2013;**144**(6):1282-91.e3. DOI: 10.1053/j.gastro.2013.02.008

[8] Sankaran SJ, Xiao AY, Wu LM, Windsor JA, Forsmark CE, Petrov MS. Frequency of progression from acute to chronic pancreatitis and risk factors: A meta-analysis. Gastroenterology. 2015;**149**(6):1490-500.e1. DOI: 10.1053/j.gastro.2015.07.066

[9] Apte MV, Pirola RC, Wilson JS. Pancreatic stellate cells: A starring role in normal and diseased pancreas. Frontiers in Physiology. 2012;**3**:344. DOI: 10.3389/fphys.2012.00344

[10] Barman KK, Premalatha G, Mohan V. Tropical chronic pancreatitis. Postgraduate Medical Journal. 2003;**79**(937):606-615. DOI: 10.1136/pmj.79.937.606

[11] Layer P, Yamamoto H, Kalthoff L, Clain JE, Bakken LJ, DiMagno EP. The different courses of early- and late-onset idiopathic and alcoholic chronic pancreatitis. Gastroenterology. 1994;**107**(5):1481-1487. DOI: 10.1016/0016-5085(94)90553-3

[12] Rockey EW. Total pancreatectomy for carcinoma: case report. Annals of Surgery. 1943;**118**(4):603-611. DOI: 10.1097/00000658-194310000-00008

[13] Ihse I, Anderson H, Andrén-Sandberg Å. Total pancreatectomy for cancer of the pancreas: Is it appropriate? World Journal of Surgery. 1996;**20**(3):288-294. DOI: 10.1007/s002689900046

[14] Puestow CB, Gillesby WJ. Retrograde surgical drainage of pancreas for chronic relapsing pancreatitis. A.M.A. Archives of Surgery. 1958;**76**(6):898-906. DOI: 10.1001/archsurg.1958.01280230022004

[15] Beger HG, Büchler M, Bittner RR, Oettinger W, Roscher R. Duodenum-preserving resection of the head of the pancreas in severe chronic pancreatitis: Early and late results. Annals of Surgery. 1989;**209**(3):273-278. DOI: 10.1097/00000658-198903000-00004

[16] Sutherland DE, Matas AJ, Najarian JS. Pancreatic islet cell transplantation. The Surgical Clinics of North America. 1978;**58**(2):365-382. DOI: 10.1016/S0039-6109(16)41490-6

[17] Zureikat AH, Moser AJ, Boone BA, Bartlett DL, Zenati M, Zeh HJ 3rd. 250 robotic pancreatic resections: Safety and feasibility. Annals of Surgery. 2013;**258**(4):554-562. DOI: 10.1097/SLA.0b013e3182a4e87c

[18] Wilson GC, Sutton JM, Salehi M, Schmulewitz N, Smith MT, Kucera S, et al. Surgical outcomes after total pancreatectomy and islet cell autotransplantation in pediatric patients. Surgery. 2013;**154**(4):777-783. DOI: 10.1016/j.surg.2013.07.003

[19] Bellin MD, Freeman ML, Gelrud A, Slivka A, Clavel A, Humar A, et al. Total pancreatectomy and islet autotransplantation in chronic pancreatitis: Recommendations from Pancreas fest. Pancreatology. 2014;**14**(1):27-35. DOI: 10.1016/j.pan.2013.10.009

[20] Garcea G, Pollard CA, Illouz S, Webb M, Metcalfe MS, Dennison AR. Patient satisfaction and cost-effectiveness following total pancreatectomy with islet cell transplantation for chronic pancreatitis. Pancreas. 2013;**42**(2):322-328. DOI: 10.1097/MPA.0b013e31826532e7

[21] Rickels MR, Robertson RP. Pancreatic islet transplantation in humans: Recent progress and future directions. Endocrine Reviews. 2019;**40**(2):631-668. DOI: 10.1210/er.2018-00154

[22] Chinnakotla S, Bellin MD, Schwarzenberg SJ, Radosevich DM, Cook M, Dunn TB, et al. Total pancreatectomy and islet autotransplantation in children for chronic pancreatitis: Indication, surgical techniques, postoperative management, and long-term outcomes. Annals of Surgery. 2014;**260**(1):56-64. DOI: 10.1097/SLA.0000000000000567

[23] Bellin MD, Kerdsirichairat T, Beilman GJ, Dunn TB, Chinnakotla S, Pruett TL, et al. Total pancreatectomy with islet autotransplantation improves quality of life in patients with refractory recurrent acute pancreatitis. Clinical Gastroenterology and Hepatology. 2016;**14**(9):1317-1323. DOI: 10.1016/j.cgh.2016.02.027

[24] Murtaugh LC, Keefe MD. Regeneration and repair of the exocrine pancreas. Annual Review of Physiology. 2015;77:229-249. DOI: 10.1146/annurev-physiol-021014-071727

[25] Bonanni P, Grazzini M, Niccolai G, Paolini D, Varone O, Bartoloni A, et al. Recommended vaccinations for asplenic and hyposplenic adult patients. Human Vaccines & Immunotherapeutics. 2017;**13**(2):359-368. DOI: 10.1080/21645515.2017.1264797

[26] Conwell DL, Lee LS, Yadav D, Longnecker DS, Miller FH, Mortele KJ, et al. American pancreatic association practice guidelines in chronic pancreatitis: Evidence-based report on diagnostic guidelines. Pancreas. 2014;**43**(8):1143-1162. DOI: 10.1097/MPA.0000000000000237

[27] Kamat R, Gupta P, Rana S. Imaging in chronic pancreatitis: State of the art

review. Indian Journal Of Radiology And Imaging. 2019;**29**(2):201-210. DOI: 10.4103/ijri.IJRI_484_18

[28] Catalano MF, Sahai A, Levy M, Romagnuolo J, Wiersema M, Brugge W, et al. EUS-based criteria for the diagnosis of chronic pancreatitis: The Rosemont classification. Gastrointestinal Endoscopy. 2009;**69**(7):1251-1261. DOI: 10.1016/j.gie.2008.07.043

[29] Berger M, Beilman GJ, Dunn T, Sutherland D, Chinnakotla S. Total pancreatectomy and islet auto-transplantation for chronic painful pancreatitis: An overview. International Journal of Transplantation Research and Medicine. 2015;**1**:014

[30] Desai CS, Stephenson DA, Khan KM, Jie T, Gruessner AC, Rilo HL, et al. Novel technique of total pancreatectomy before autologous islet transplants in chronic pancreatitis patients. Journal of the American College of Surgeons. 2011;**213**(6):e29-e34. DOI: 10.1016/j.jamcollsurg.2011.09.008

[31] Ricordi C, Lacy PE, Scharp DW. Automated islet isolation from human pancreas. Diabetes. 1989;**38**(Suppl. 1):140-142. DOI: 10.2337/diab.38.1.s140

[32] Cantarelli E, Piemonti L. Alternative transplantation sites for pancreatic islet grafts. Current Diabetes Reports. 2011;**11**(5):364-374. DOI: 10.1007/s11892-011-0216-9

[33] Galvani CA, Rodriguez Rilo H, Samamé J, Porubsky M, Rana A, Gruessner RW. Fully robotic-assisted technique for total pancreatectomy with an autologous islet transplant in chronic pancreatitis patients: Results of a first series. Journal of the American College of Surgeons. 2014;**218**(3):e73-e78. DOI: 10.1016/j.jamcollsurg.2013.12.006

[34] Berger M, Bellin MD, Kirchner V, Schwarzenberg SJ, Chinnakotla S. Laparoscopic-assisted versus open total pancreatectomy and islet autotransplantation: A case-matched study of pediatric patients. Journal of Pediatric Surgery. 2020;**55**(3):558-563. DOI: 10.1016/j.jpedsurg.2019.10.007

[35] Weng Y, Chen M, Gemenetzis G, Shi Y, Ying X, Deng X, et al. Robotic-assisted versus open total pancreatectomy: A propensity score-matched study. Hepatobiliary Surgery and Nutrition. 2020;**9**(6):759-770. DOI: 10.21037/hbsn.2020.03.19

[36] Gruessner R, Cercone R, Galvani C, Rana A, Porubsky M, Gruessner A, et al. Results of open and robot-assisted pancreatectomies with autologous islet transplantations: Treating chronic pancreatitis and preventing surgically induced diabetes. Transplantation Proceedings. 2014;**46**:1978-1979. DOI: 10.1016/j.transproceed.2014.06.005

[37] Scholten L, Klompmaker S, Van Hilst J, Annecchiarico MM, Balzano G, Casadei R, et al. Outcomes after minimally invasive versus open total pancreatectomy: A pan-European propensity score matched study. Annals of Surgery. 2023;**277**(2):313-320. DOI: 10.1097/SLA.0000000000005075

[38] Forlenza GP, Chinnakotla S, Schwarzenberg SJ, Cook M, Radosevich DM, Manchester C, et al. Near-euglycemia can be achieved safely in pediatric total pancreatectomy islet autotransplant recipients using an adapted intravenous insulin infusion protocol. Diabetes Technology & Therapeutics. 2014;**16**(11):706-713. DOI: 10.1089/dia.2014.0061

[39] Naziruddin B, Kanak MA, Chang CA, Takita M, Lawrence MC, Dennison AR, et al. Improved outcomes

of islet autotransplant after total pancreatectomy by combined blockade of IL-1β and TNFα. American Journal of Transplantation. 2018;**18**(9):2322-2329. DOI: 10.1111/ajt.14961

[40] Chinnakotla S, Radosevich DM, Dunn TB, Bellin MD, Freeman ML, Schwarzenberg SJ, et al. Long-term outcomes of total pancreatectomy and islet auto transplantation for hereditary/genetic pancreatitis. Journal of the American College of Surgeons. 2014;**218**(4):530-543. DOI: 10.1016/j.jamcollsurg.2013.12.037

[41] Morgan KA, Lancaster WP, Owczarski SM, Wang H, Borckardt J, Adams DB. Patient selection for Total pancreatectomy with islet autotransplantation in the surgical Management of Chronic Pancreatitis. Journal of the American College of Surgeons. 2018;**226**(4):446-451. DOI: 10.1016/j.jamcollsurg.2017.12.018

[42] Wilson GC, Sutton JM, Abbott DE, Smith MT, Lowy AM, Matthews JB, et al. Long-term outcomes after total pancreatectomy and islet cell autotransplantation: Is it a durable operation? Annals of Surgery. 2014;**260**(4):659-667. DOI: 10.1097/SLA.0000000000000920

[43] Sutherland DE, Radosevich DM, Bellin MD, Hering BJ, Beilman GJ, Dunn TB, et al. Total pancreatectomy and islet autotransplantation for chronic pancreatitis. Journal of the American College of Surgeons. 2012;**214**(4):409-424. DOI: 10.1016/j.jamcollsurg.2011.12.040

[44] Coluzzi M, Takita M, Saracino G, Rub Hakim Mohammed A, Darden CM, Testa G, et al. Improved quality of life among chronic pancreatitis patients undergoing total pancreatectomy with islet autotransplantation—Single center experience with large cohort of patients. Transplant International. 2023;**36**:11409. DOI: 10.3389/ti.2023.11409

[45] Sutton JM, Schmulewitz N, Sussman JJ, Smith M, Kurland JE, Brunner JE, et al. Total pancreatectomy and islet cell autotransplantation as a means of treating patients with genetically linked pancreatitis. Surgery. 2010;**148**(4):676-685. DOI: 10.1016/j.surg.2010.07.043

Section 4

Upper Gastrointestinal Surgical Oncology

Chapter 8

Robotic Total and Near-Total (98%) Gastrectomy

Beniamino Pascotto, Martine Goergen and Juan Santiago Azagra

Abstract

Minimally invasive techniques for gastrectomy have evolved significantly since the first laparoscopic distal gastrectomy in 1991. However, laparoscopic total gastrectomy (LTG) remains technically challenging due to the complexity of lymphadenectomy and esophagojejunostomy reconstruction. Our team pioneered LTG in 1993 and has since advanced minimally invasive approaches, including the laparoscopic near-total gastrectomy and, more recently, a fully robotic technique. The robotic approach enhances surgical precision, facilitating D2-lymphadenectomy, and optimizes hand-sewn alimentary tract reconstruction. The procedure is performed using four robotic ports and a liver retractor; there is no laparoscopic assistance. The en bloc lymphadenectomy is clockwise and follows a structured sequence, ensuring oncologic safety. The reconstruction phase, particularly esophagojejunostomy, remains the most significant technical hurdle. Our team utilizes a hand-sewn barbed suture technique for anastomosis, improving reproducibility and reducing operative time. Near-total gastrectomy follows a similar approach, preserving a minimal gastric stump. Robotic surgery addresses laparoscopic limitations by enhancing precision, reducing anastomotic tension, and streamlining suturing. The reproducibility of robotic hand-sewn anastomosis and its superior outcomes may establish it as the preferred technique for total and near-total gastrectomy, promoting wider adoption in gastric cancer treatment.

Keywords: robotic total gastrectomy, robotic near-total gastrectomy, Azagra's anastomosis, esophagojejunostomy, gastrojejunostomy, real robotic surgery

1. Introduction

Since Kitano performed the first laparoscopic distal gastrectomy (LDG) in 1991 and subsequently described it in 1994 [1], the minimally invasive approach has become the gold standard for distal gastrectomies [2–6].

However, the adoption of a minimally invasive technique for total gastrectomy (TG) has been more challenging due to the technical complexity of the procedure.

Our team first reported laparoscopic TG for gastric cancer in 1993 [7]. Since then, multiple studies have demonstrated the feasibility and safety of LTG for early-stage gastric cancer and, more recently, for advanced disease [8–18].

The limited uptake of laparoscopic TG is primarily attributed to two critical challenges: achieving an adequate lymphadenectomy, which is essential for oncologic safety, and performing the esophagojejunostomy, which is crucial for surgical safety. Both factors directly influence patient prognosis [19–23].

D2 lymphadenectomy is the standard of care for gastric cancer [24, 25].

Laparoscopic-assisted TG remains the most commonly performed approach, as the esophagojejunostomy is typically constructed using a circular stapler through a mini-laparotomy [26–31].

Described in 1980, Near-Total Gastrectomy (NTG) aims to reduce the anastomosis-related complications of TG without affecting its oncological radicality [32–34]. Our group described in 2014 the laparoscopic approach for NTG [35, 36].

Since 2018, we have performed both TG and NTG using a Real Robotic Approach. There are no laparoscopic assisting ports (except for the liver retractor, which is fixed).

Robotic surgical platforms have addressed many of the technical limitations associated with laparoscopic TG, improving both lymphadenectomy and reconstruction, thereby enhancing the feasibility and safety of the procedure.

Our team described the Azagra's anastomosis for alimentary tract reconstruction during minimally invasive TG and NTG [37–39]. The robotic approach facilitates precise and minimal mobilization of the esophageal stump, thereby reducing anastomotic tension and contributing to improved surgical outcomes [20–22, 38–41]. The implementation of barbed sutures in robotic hand-sewn esophagojejunostomy has further streamlined the procedure by reducing operative time and technical complexity while achieving outcomes that are comparable to or superior to conventional non-barbed hand-sewn techniques.

Robotic surgical platforms optimize lymphadenectomy by enabling enhanced precision in complex dissections. This advantage, combined with the reproducibility of hand-sewn esophagojejunostomy, establishes robotic-assisted minimally invasive TG and NTG as a promising standard approach. Although hand-sewn anastomosis presents a steep learning curve, the integration of robotic technology has the potential to mitigate this challenge, promoting wider adoption of the technique. Ultimately, robotic hand-sewn anastomosis may emerge as the preferred approach for alimentary tract reconstruction following TG and NTG, offering superior oncologic and surgical outcomes [42].

2. Surgical technique

2.1 Patient installation

The robotic platform adopted is the da Vinci Xi, Intuitive. The patient is in anti-Trendelenburg position of 18° and right rotation of 4°. The port placements consist of four robotic ports, three of 8 mm and one of 12 mm. The procedure is performed with two "right hands," which means that the camera is in the arm number two. From the right to the left the first port is a 8 mm robotic port for the bipolar grasper; the second port is a 8 mm robotic port for the camera; the third port is a 12 mm robotic port for the monopolar scissors, the advanced energy device (Vessel Sealer, da Vinci Xi®, Intuitive), the 60-mm SureForm™ robotic stapler (da Vinci Xi®, Intuitive); the fourth port is a 8 mm robotic port for the Cadiere grasper. An additional 5 mm laparoscopic port is put in the right upper quadrant for the liver retractor. The 12 mm port is also used in order to introduce a little gauze and the stitches by the bedside assistant (**Figure 1**).

2.2 Dissection time

The "en bloc" lymphadenectomy is clockwise in the following order of lymph node groups: 4d, 6, 5, 8a, 12a, 9, 11p, 7, 1 (group 3 goes together). The second part is anticlockwise in the following order of lymph node groups: 4sb, 4sa, 2 (**Figure 2**).

The procedure begins with the opening of the gastrocolic ligament, maintaining a distance of 5 cm lateral to the gastroepiploic arcade to ensure the removal of all lymph nodes in group 4d, which are located along the arcade (**Figures 3–5**). While staying 5 cm lateral to the arcade, this dissection continues downward to reach the Gastrocolic Intrafascial Space (GIS). This is an avascular space filled with connective and adipose tissue, located between the posterior surface of the greater omentum and the transverse mesocolon. By opening this space, access is gained to the right gastroepiploic vessels, completing the lymphadenectomy of group 6 (**Figures 6** and **7**). The gastroepiploic vein is divided with clips close to the head of the pancreas, just before the confluence

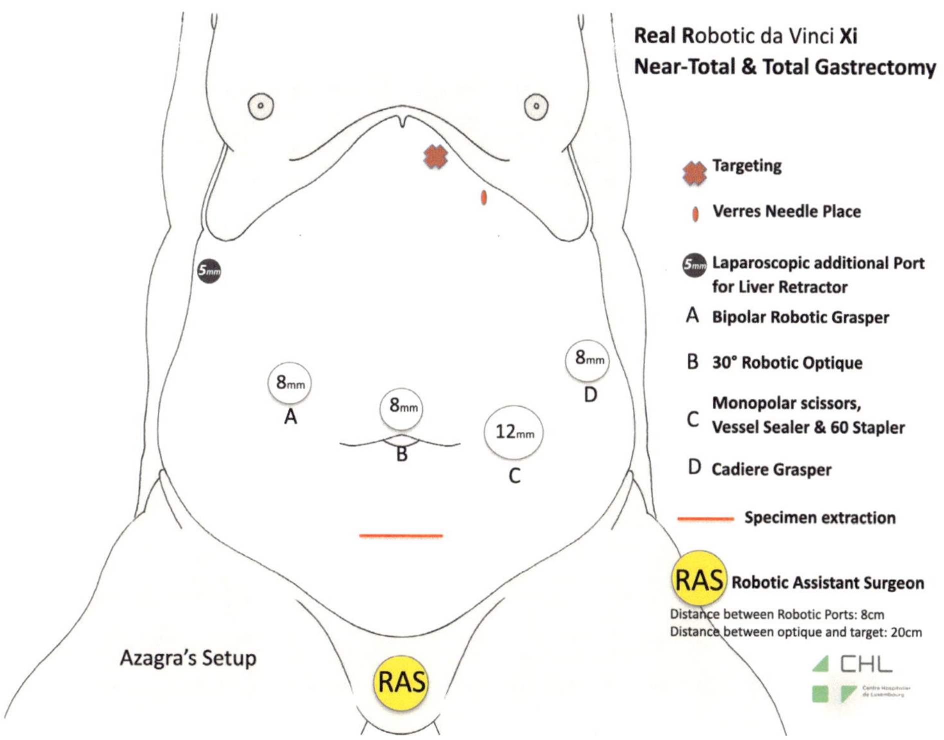

Figure 1.
Patient installation and ports position.

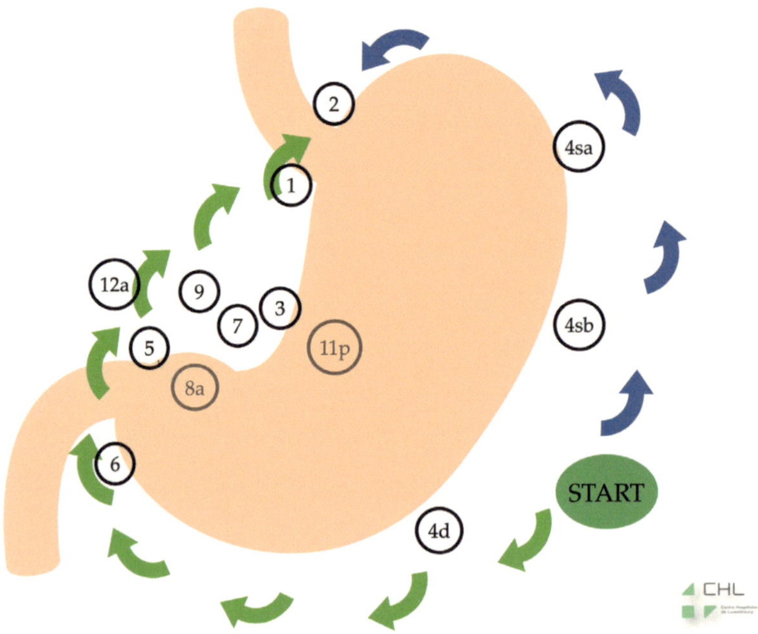

Figure 2.
Steps of lymphadenectomy; starting point (START); first step clockwise (green arrow); second step anticlockwise (blue arrow).

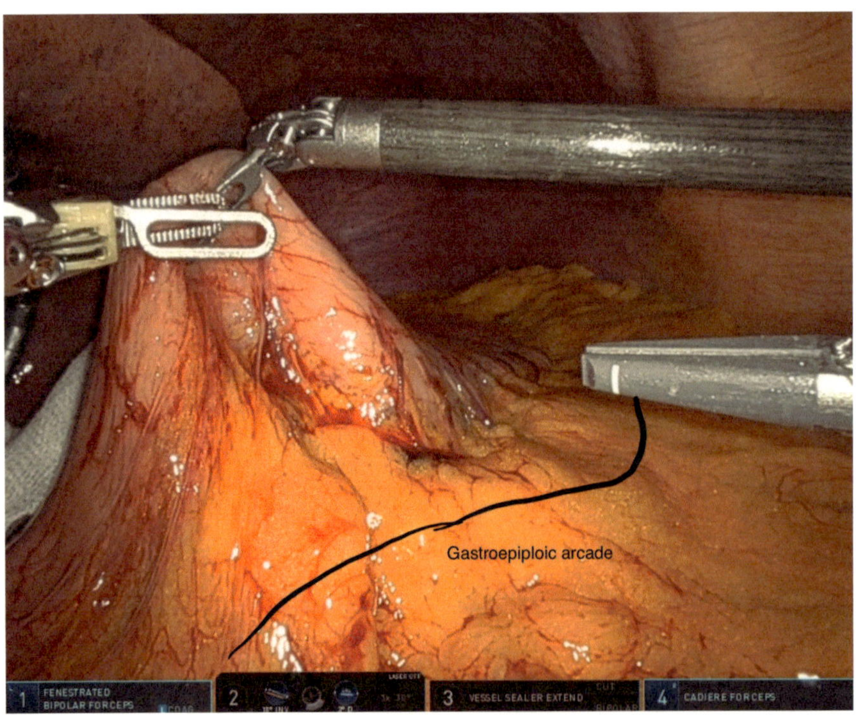

Figure 3.
Gastroepiploic arcade with lymph nodes group 4d.

DOI: http://dx.doi.org/10.5772/intechopen.1010625

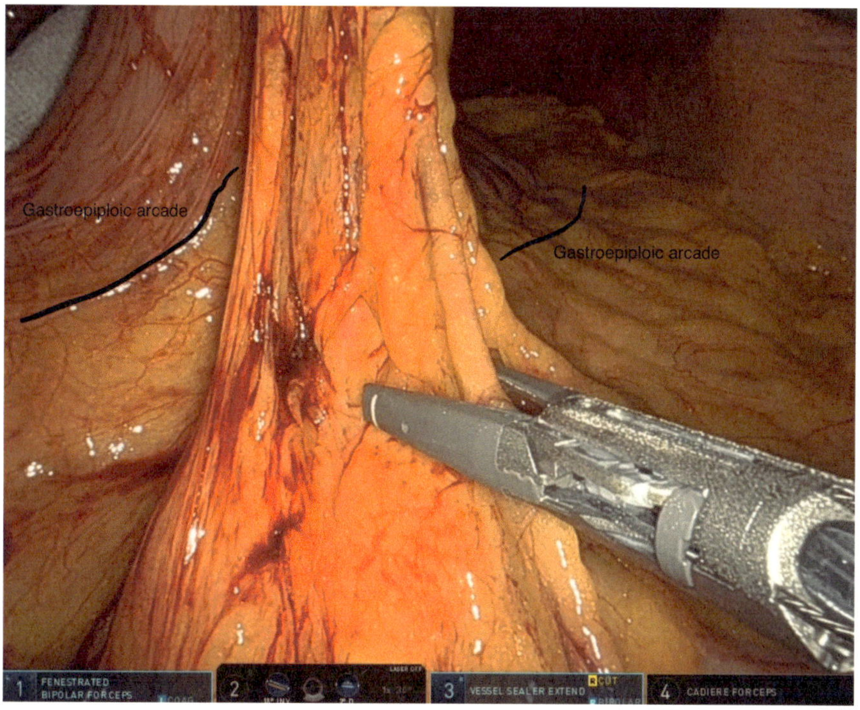

Figure 4.
Opening of the gastrocolic ligament and access to the retro-gastric cavity.

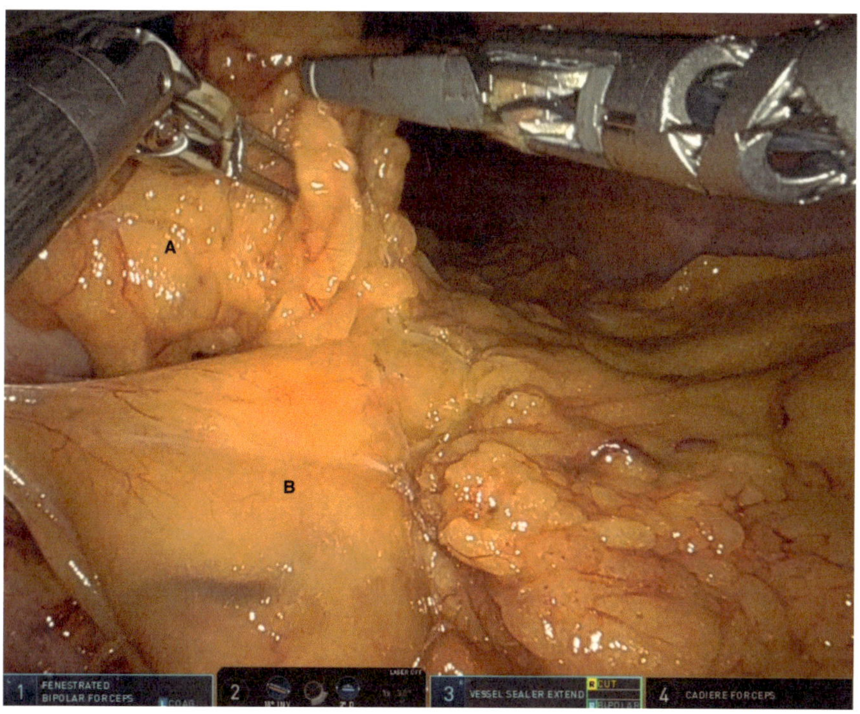

Figure 5.
Lymph nodes group 4d (A); transverse mesocolon (B).

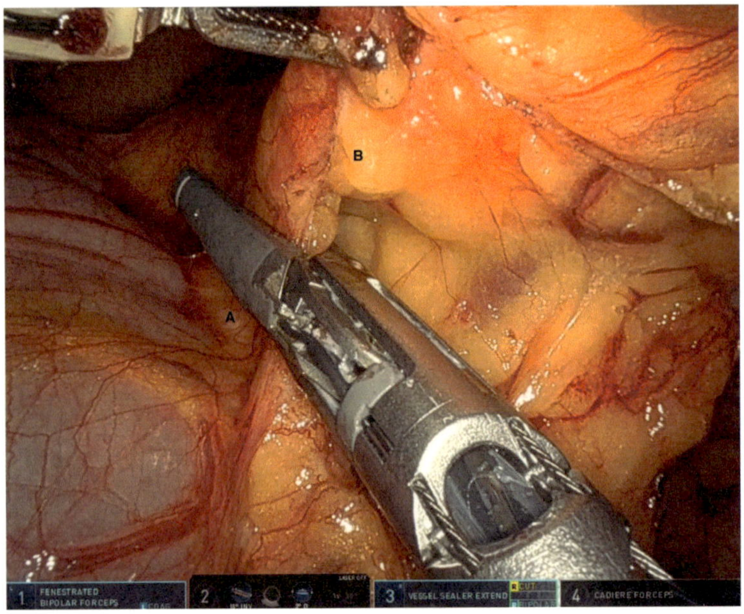

Figure 6.
Head of the pancreas (A); lymph nodes group 6 (B).

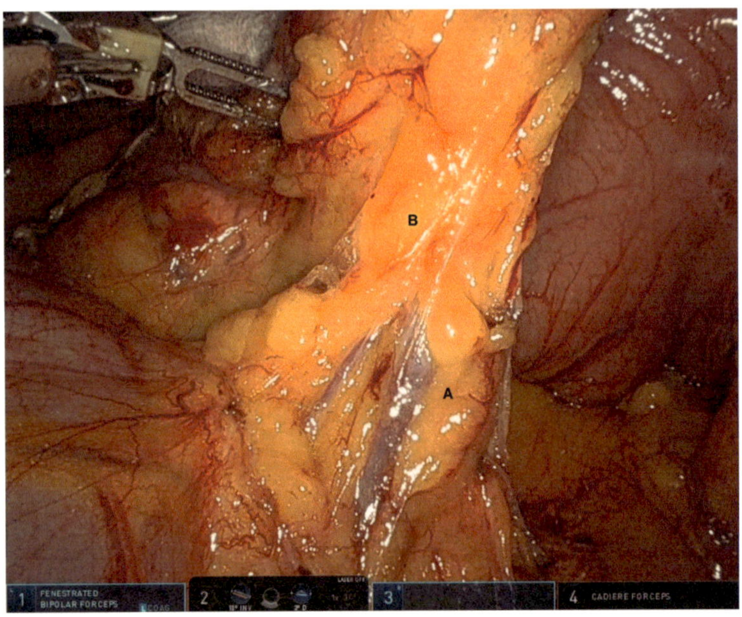

Figure 7.
Middle colic vessels (A); lymph nodes group 6 (B).

with the Henle trunk (**Figure 8**). The gastroduodenal artery is visualized on the anterior face of the pancreas. This artery is followed downward to its bifurcation into the right gastroepiploic artery and the superior pancreaticoduodenal artery. The right gastroepiploic artery is then divided with clips at its origin (**Figures 9** and **10**). The

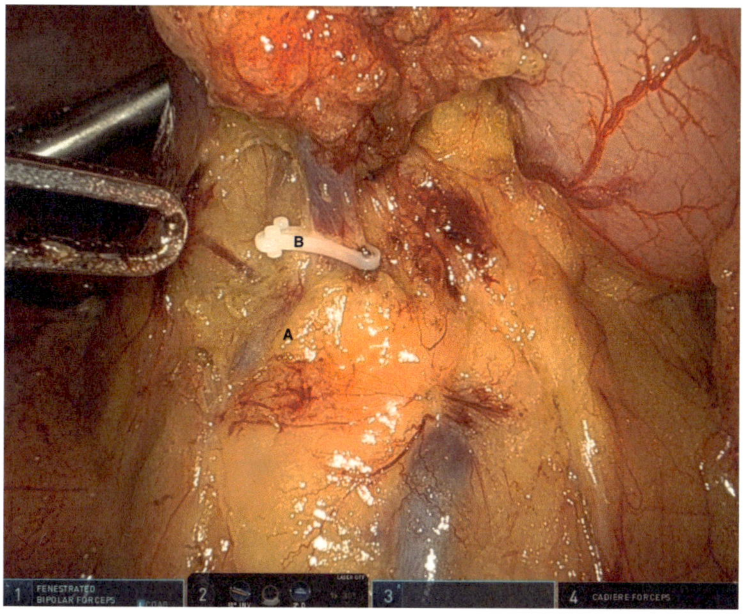

Figure 8.
Middle colic vein (A); right gastroepiploic vein (B).

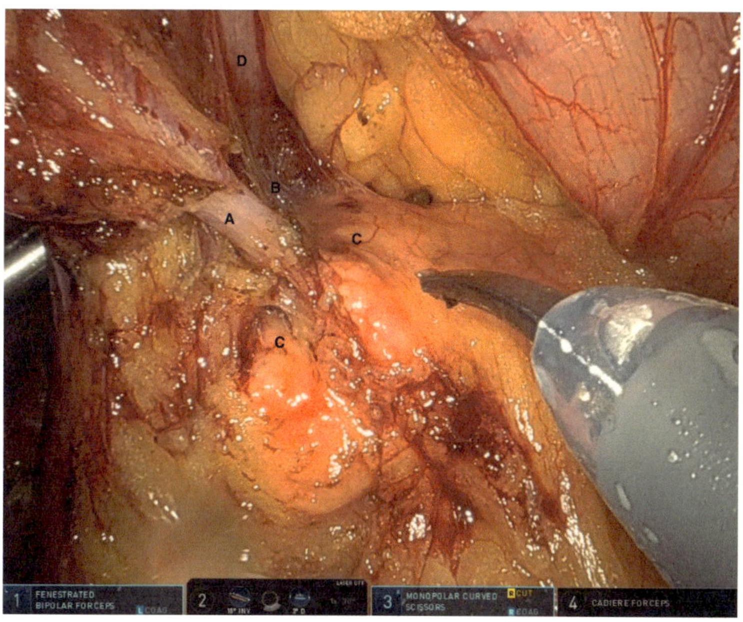

Figure 9.
Right gastroepiploic artery (A); gastroduodenal artery (B); pancreas (C).

pancreaticoduodenal fascia (PDF) is derived from the posterior layer of the dorsal mesogastrium. This fascia corresponds to the cellular-lymphatic tissue covering the head of the pancreas and is dissected following a virtual line from the origin of the right gastroepiploic vessels to the duodenum, along a trajectory targeting the gallbladder

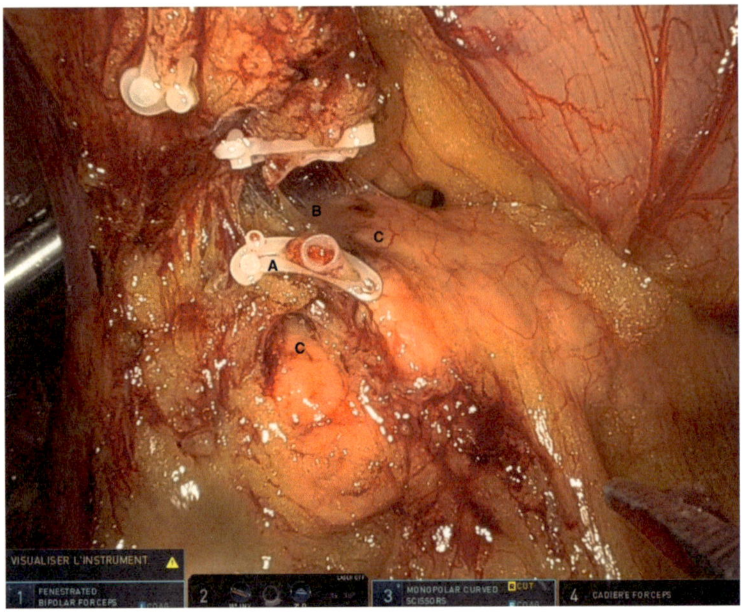

Figure 10.
Right gastroepiploic artery stump after transection (A); gastroduodenal artery (B); pancreas (C).

(**Figures 11–13**). This ensures the removal of all infrapyloric lymph nodes. The lymph nodes group 5 is dissected on the superior margin of the pylorus, opening the hepatogastric ligament along the stomach (**Figure 14**). The dissection continues medial to lateral, reaching the first part of the duodenum (**Figure 15**). This is then transected

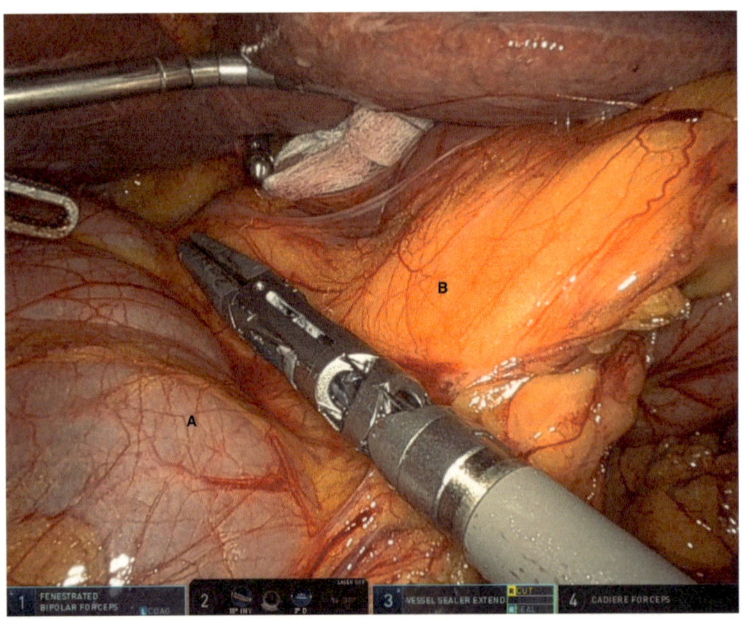

Figure 11.
Transverse colon (A); lymph nodes group 6 (B).

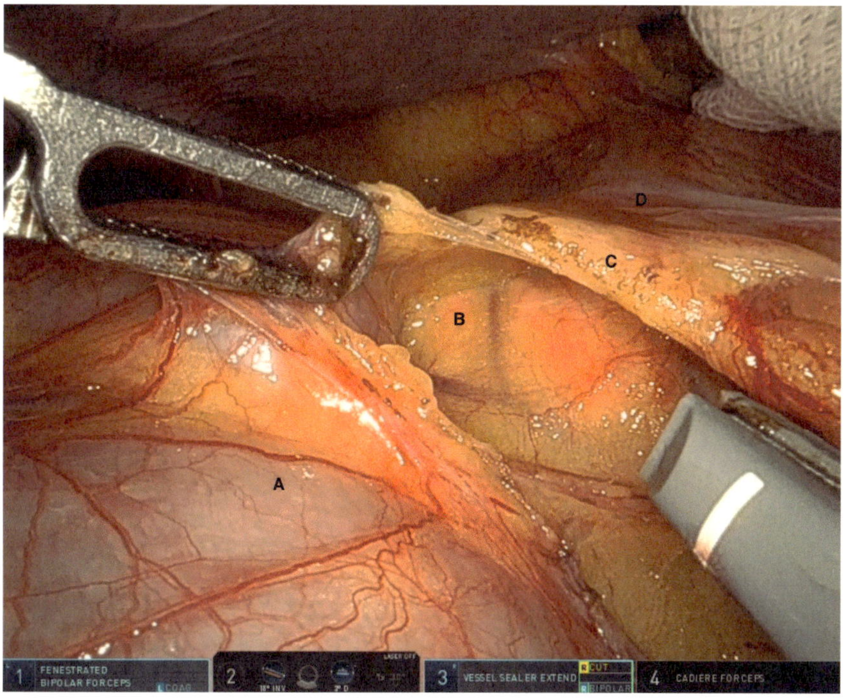

Figure 12.
Transverse colon (A); head of the pancreas (B); greater omentum (C); duodenum (D).

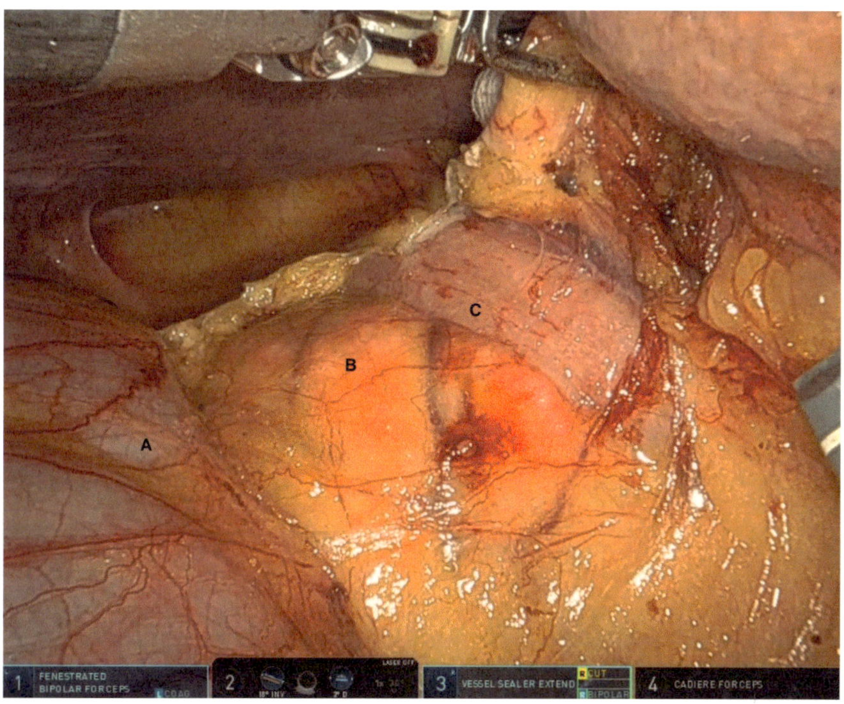

Figure 13.
Transverse colon (A); head of the pancreas (B); duodenum (C).

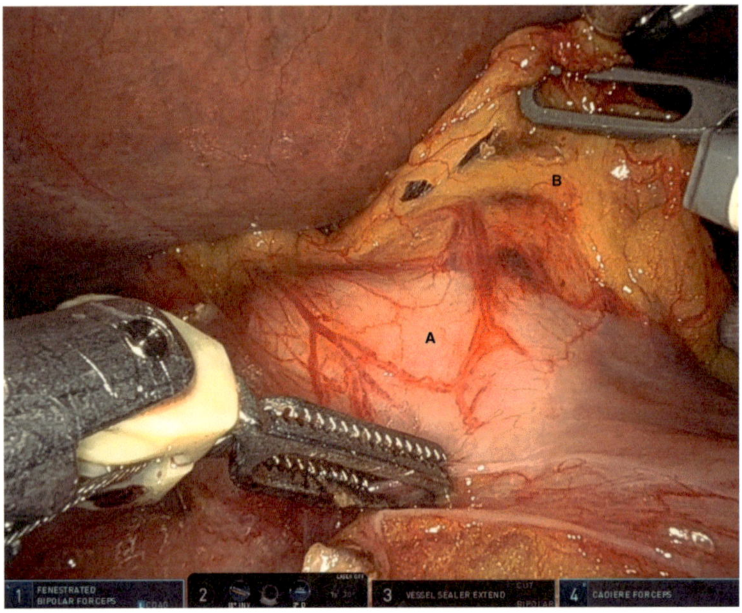

Figure 14.
Pylorus (A); lymph nodes group 5 (B).

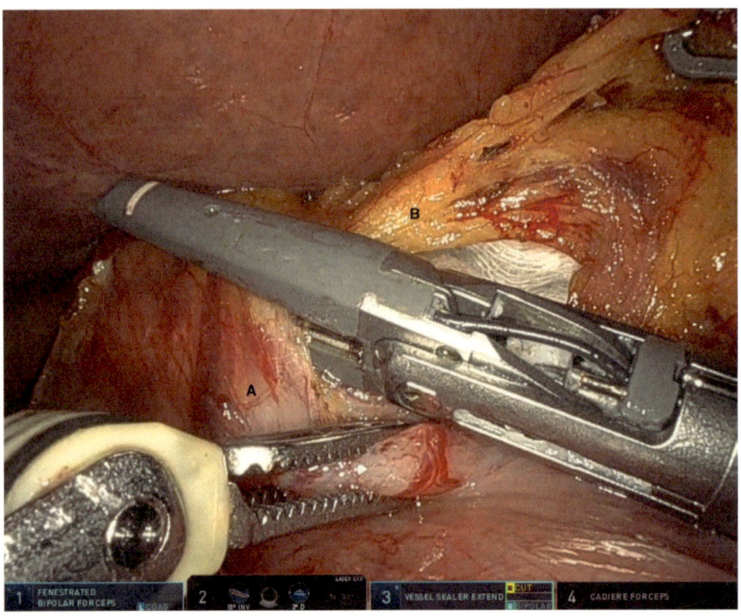

Figure 15.
Pylorus and supra-pyloric dissection targeting the first duodenum (A); lymph nodes group 5 (B).

using a 60-mm SureForm™ robotic stapler (da Vinci Xi®, Intuitive) with a blue cartridge, inserted through arm 3. The stapler is positioned thanks to its articulation (**Figures 16** and **17**).

The stomach is then retracted to the patient's left side to facilitate access to the superior margin of the pancreas (**Figure 18**). The lymphadenectomy of groups 11p

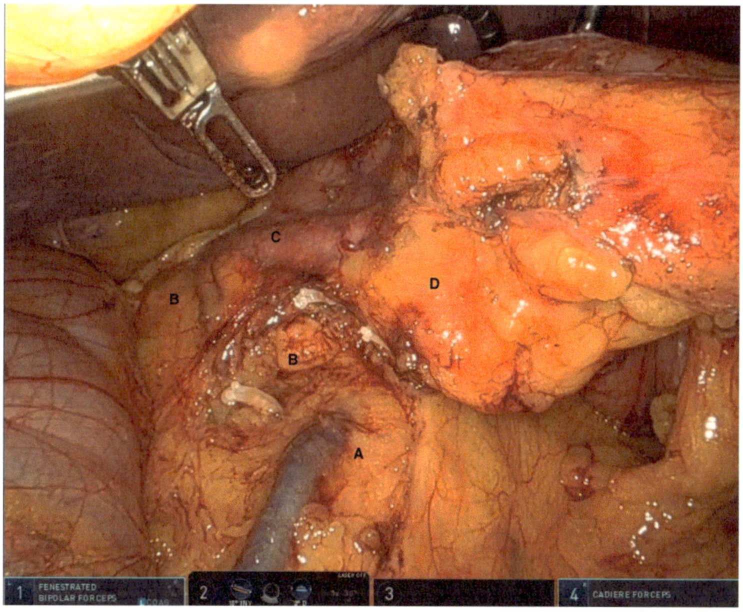

Figure 16.
Middle colic vein (A); pancreas (B); duodenum (C); lymph nodes group 6 (D).

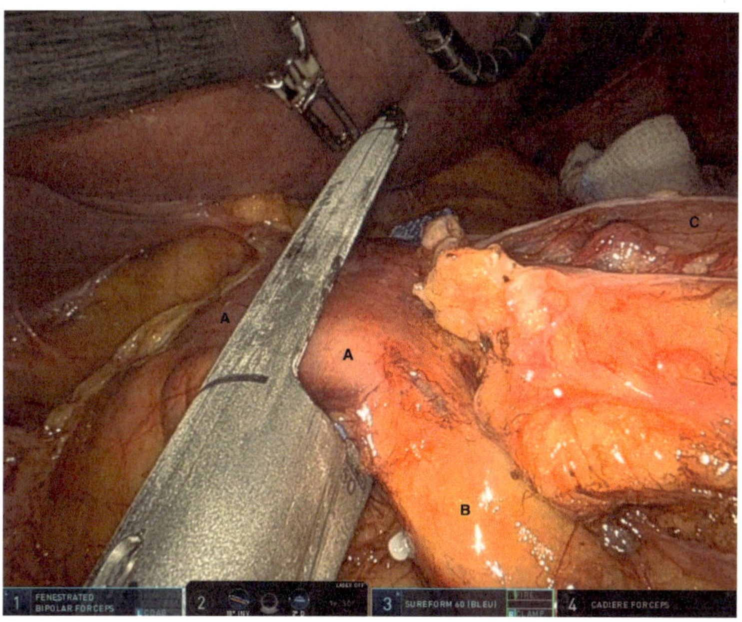

Figure 17.
Duodenum (A); lymph nodes group 6 (B).

and 8a begins with the dissection of the parietal peritoneum covering the anterior surface of the superior margin pancreas at the level of the bifurcation between the common hepatic artery and the splenic artery (**Figure 19**). During this dissection, the left gastric vein is quickly encountered, except in cases of anatomical variations,

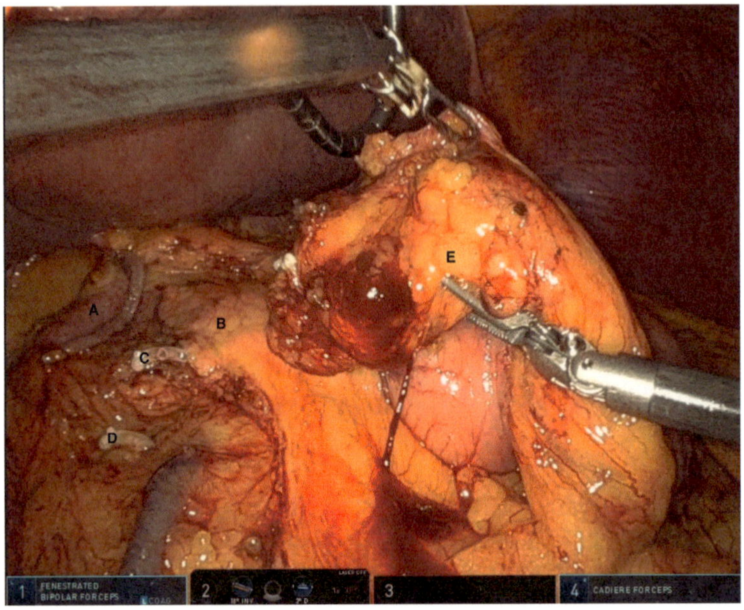

Figure 18.
Duodenum (A); pancreas (B); right gastroepiploic artery (C); right gastroepiploic vein (D); Lymph nodes group 6 (E).

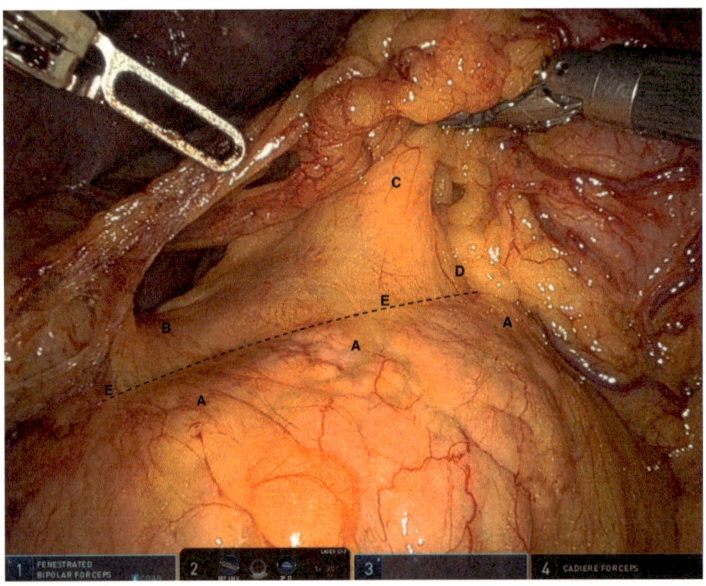

Figure 19.
Superior margin of the pancreas (A); lymph nodes group 8a (B); lymph nodes group 7 (C); lymph nodes group 11p (D); dissection plane between the pancreas and the lymph nodes groups 11p and 8a (E).

just before its connection to the portal vein. The left gastric vein is then divided with clips (**Figure 20**). The dissection continues rightward along the pancreas to the gastroduodenal artery and then superiorly to the junction between the common hepatic artery and the gastroduodenal artery. The group 8a lymph node packet is then

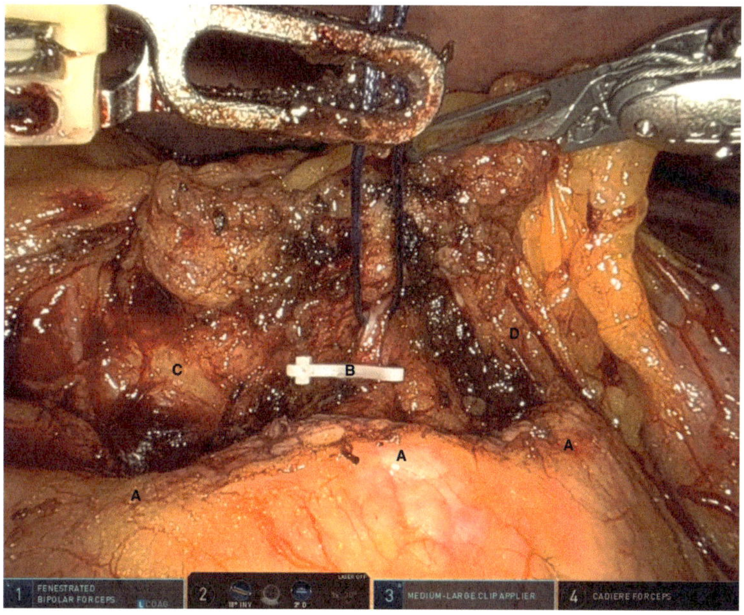

Figure 20.
Pancreas (A); left gastric vein (B); lymph nodes group 8a (C); lymph nodes group 11p (D).

lifted to access the plane between the common hepatic artery and the superior border of the pancreas. Dissecting this space leads directly to the anterolateral left border of the portal vein (**Figure 21**). The common hepatic artery is then dissected from the group 8a lymph node packet and secured with an elastic loop to facilitate traction and

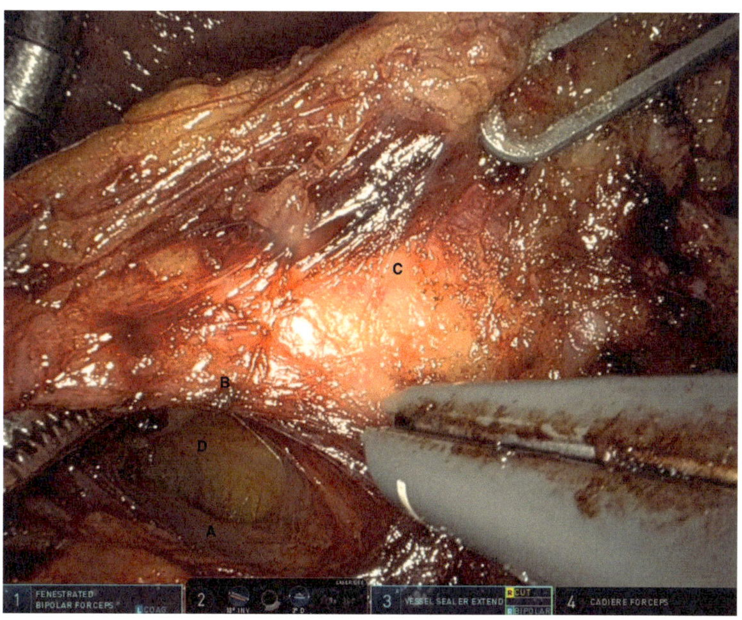

Figure 21.
Portal vein (A); common hepatic artery (B); lymph nodes group 8a (C); lymph nodes group 12a (D).

exposure for the lymphadenectomy of groups 12a and 9 (**Figure 22**). The dissection of group 12a is performed both above and below the hepatic artery, following the left lateral border of the hepatic artery and the portal vein. In most cases, the right gastric artery is encountered and divided at this point. The dissection of group 12a continues upward to the hepatic hilum. The lymph node packet is then retracted to the patient's left side, and with downward traction of the common hepatic artery, the "en bloc" lymphadenectomy of group 9 is performed, extending the dissection to the base of the right diaphragmatic crus (**Figure 23**). Lymph nodes group 11p is dissected "en bloc" on the superior margin of the pancreas, starting at the bifurcation between the splenic artery and the hepatic artery. The dissection then moves upward to group 7 at the emergence of the left gastric artery, which is secured with a Vicryl suture for exposure and then divided with clips (**Figure 24**). The dissection continues superiorly to the convergence of the diaphragmatic crura, moving toward the right crura to complete the right-side lymphadenectomy by removing the group 1 lymph nodes (**Figures** 25 and **26**). Returning to the greater curvature, the dissection of the greater omentum continues, maintaining a 5 cm lateral distance from the gastroepiploic arcade to retrieve the lymph nodes of groups 4sb and 4sa (**Figures** 27 and **28**). This dissection extends to the left diaphragmatic crura to begin the lymphadenectomy of group 2 using a lateral-to-medial approach. The group 2 lymphadenectomy is completed by returning anteriorly with a medial-to-lateral approach.

In an NTG, the lymphadenectomies of groups 1 and 2 are performed while carefully preserving the phrenoesophageal membrane, ensuring adequate vascularization of the remaining 1 cm of the gastric stump preserved for the reconstruction.

In a TG, the esophagus is transected using a 60-mm SureForm™ robotic stapler (da Vinci Xi®, Intuitive) with a blue cartridge, inserted through arm 3, positioned thanks to its articulation.

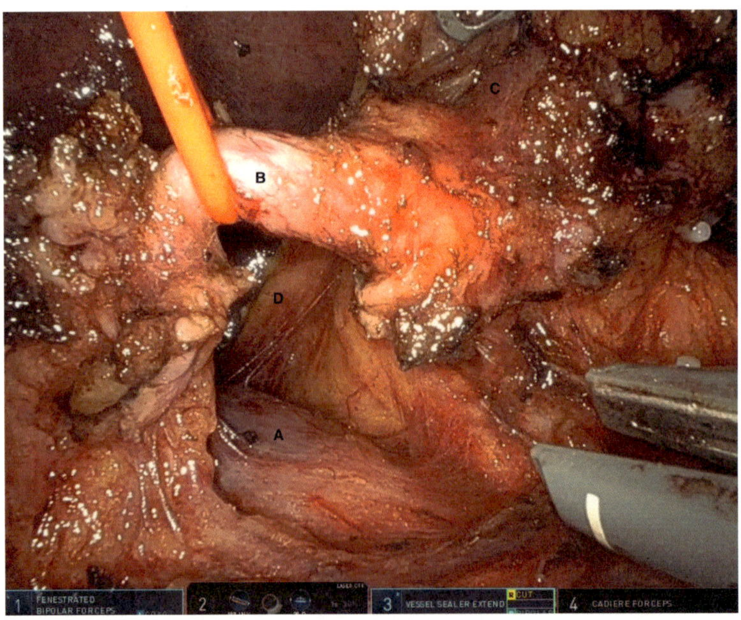

Figure 22.
Portal vein (A); common hepatic artery under loop to achieve a better exposition (B); lymph nodes group 8a (C); lymph nodes group 12a (D).

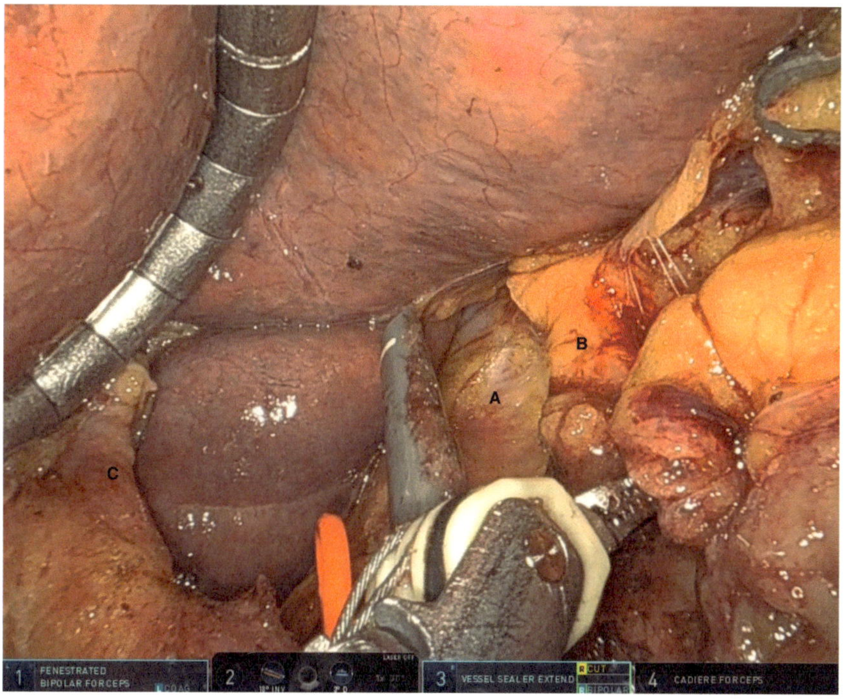

Figure 23.
Right diaphragmatic crus (A); lymph nodes group 9 (B).

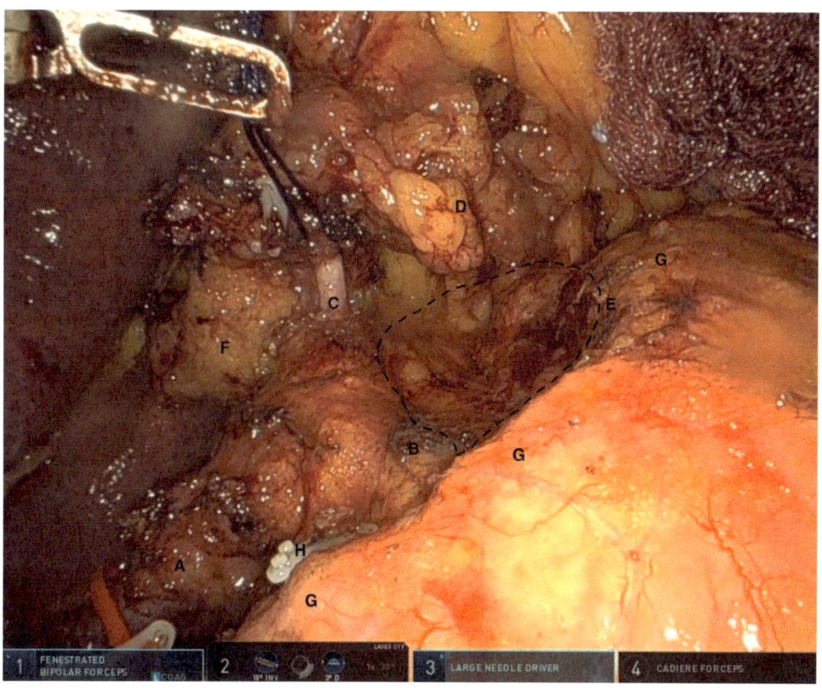

Figure 24.
Common hepatic artery (A); splenic artery (B); left gastric artery (C); lymph nodes group 11p (D); dotted line showing the area of dissection of lymph nodes group 11p (E); lymph nodes group 9 (F); pancreas (G).

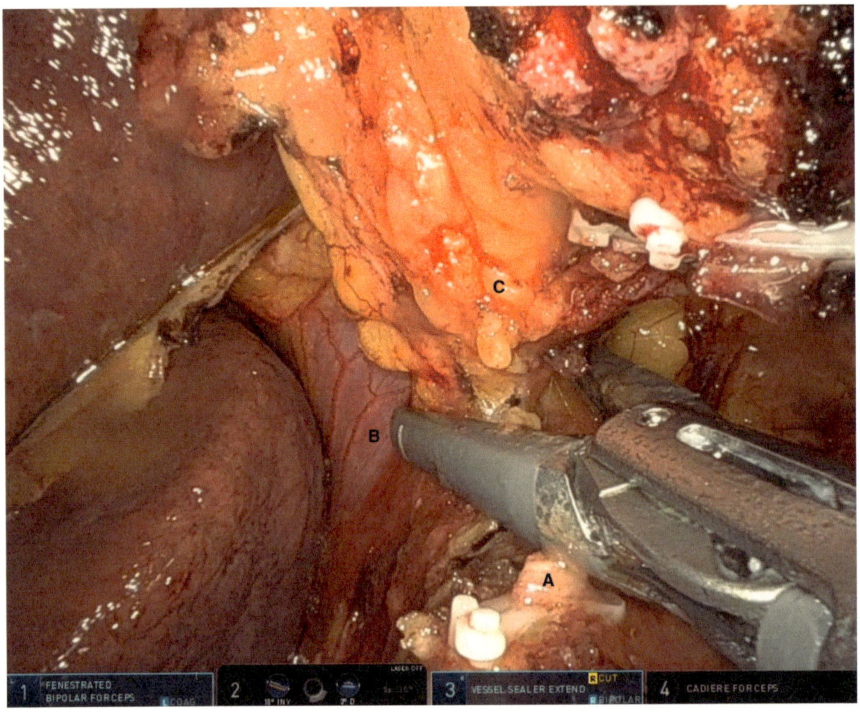

Figure 25.
Left gastric artery (A); right diaphragmatic crus (B); lymph nodes group 7 (C).

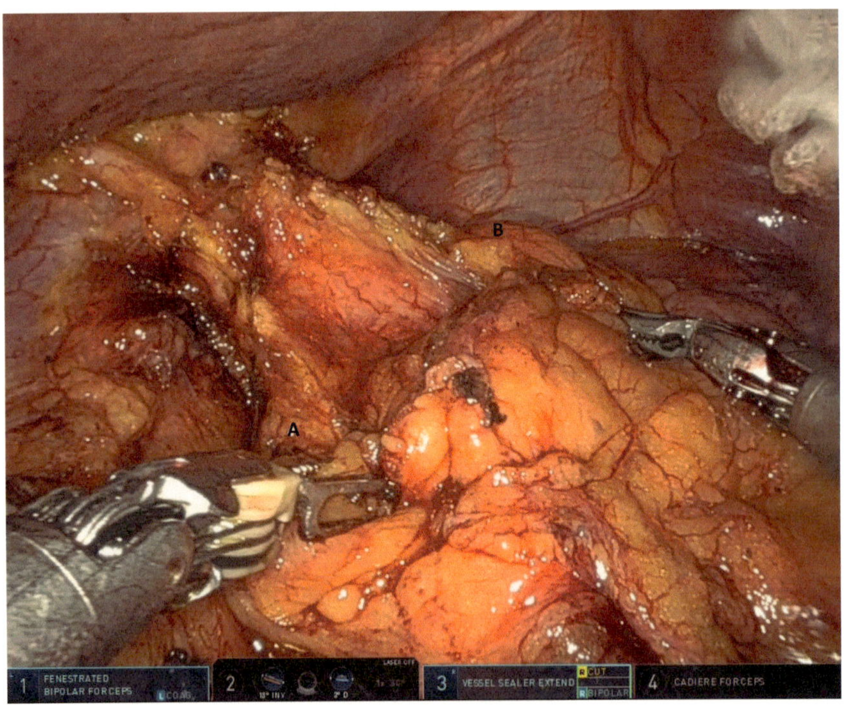

Figure 26.
Lymph nodes group 1 (A); lymph nodes group 2 (B).

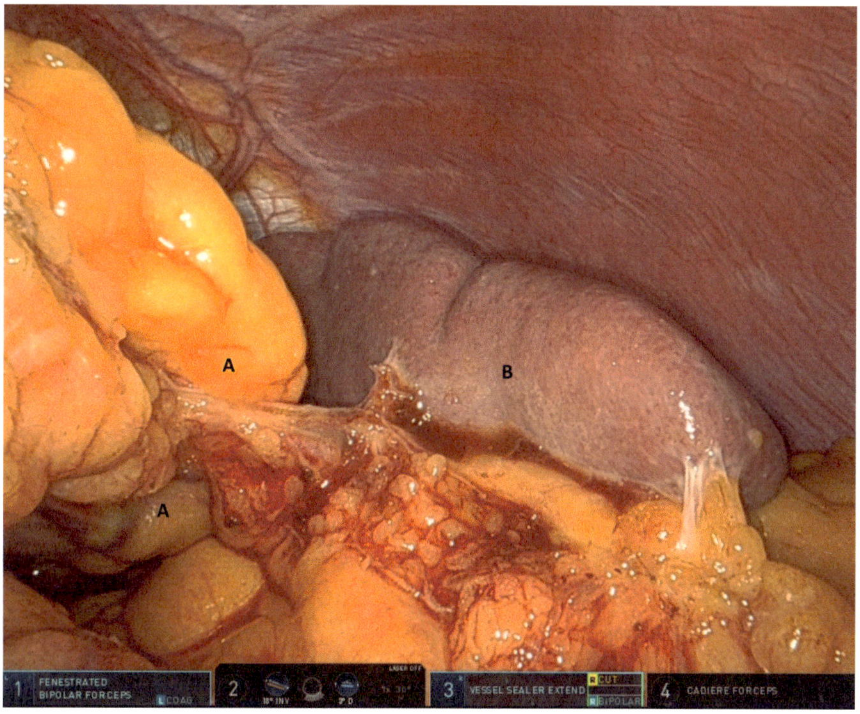

Figure 27.
Lymph nodes group 4sb (A); spleen (B).

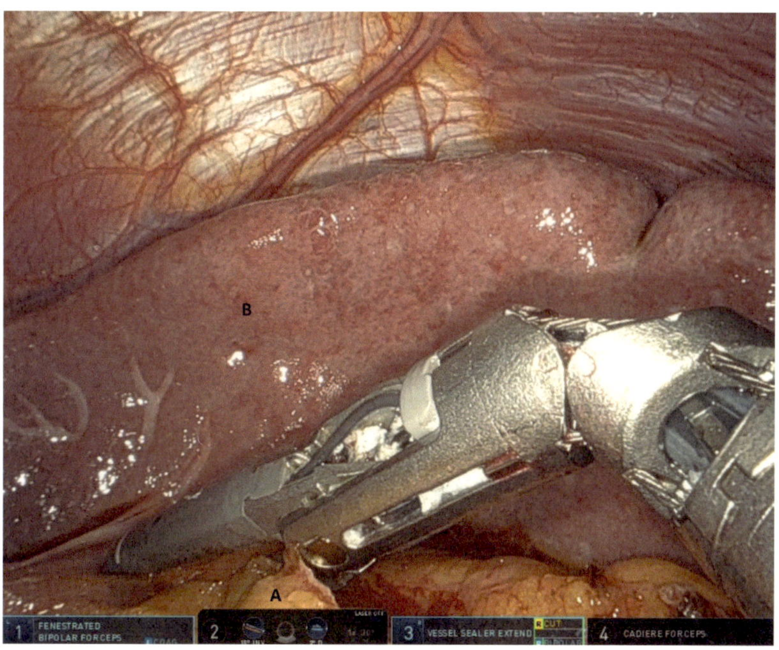

Figure 28.
Lymph nodes group 4sa; spleen (B).

In a NTG, the stomach is transected using a 60-mm SureForm™ robotic stapler (da Vinci Xi®, Intuitive) with a blue cartridge, inserted through arm 3, positioned thanks to its articulation, with two staple loads—one transversal and one vertical to ensure preservation of a 1 cm gastric stump for the anastomosis.

2.3 Reconstruction

2.3.1 Gastro-Jejunostomy

The reconstruction phase is the second major challenge of this procedure and the main reason why laparoscopy has had such low adoption in TG. Our team performs this anastomosis using the Azagra technique.

The anastomosis is performed as an end-to-side, hand-sewn technique utilizing two continuous suture layers—posterior and anterior—employing a 15-cm, 3/0 absorbable barbed V-Loc® suture (Covidien, USA).

The esophagus is advanced into the abdominal cavity using a 42-Fr endoluminal bougie, maintained under gentle pressure by the anesthesiologist. The construction of the posterior layer of the anastomosis is initiated with a running 3/0 absorbable barbed suture, beginning at the left extremity of the esophageal staple line. This suture incorporates the full thickness of both the esophageal and jejunal walls, ensuring inclusion of the esophageal staple line (**Figure 29**).

The adequate vascularization of the esophageal (or gastric, in the case of NTG) stump is confirmed with an indocyanine green test (**Figure 30**).

The esophagotomy is always performed following the completion of the posterior layer to ensure that the enterotomy conforms to the suture rather than the reverse, thereby facilitating the suturing process. The anesthesiologist advances the bougie while maintaining gentle pressure, and under this tension, the esophagotomy is

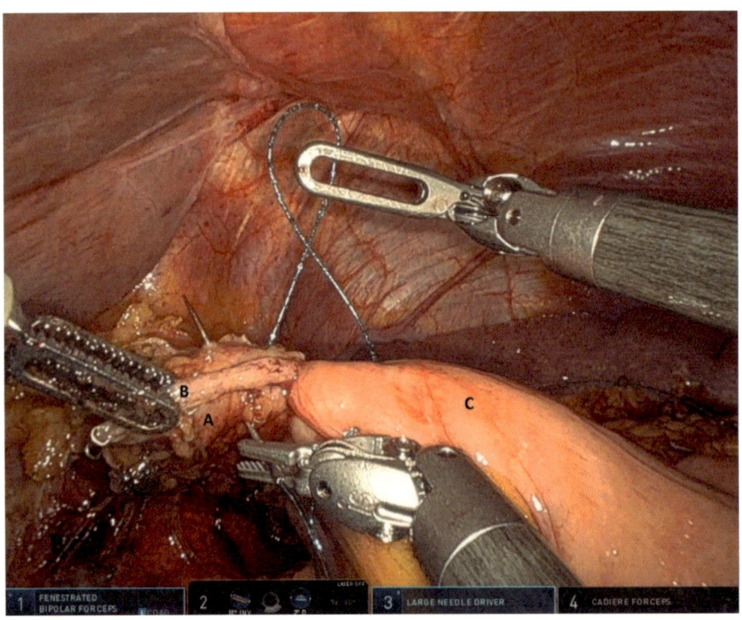

Figure 29.
Gastric stump during NTG (A); stapled line (B); jejunum (C).

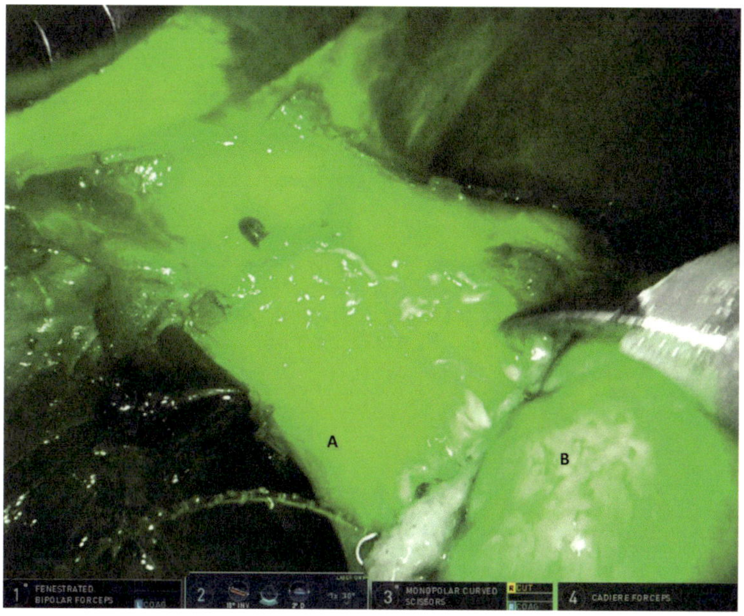

Figure 30.
Indocyanine green check of the gastric stump (A) and jejunum (B) during NTG.

created using a monopolar device. A 42-Fr bougie is utilized to calibrate the esophagotomy (**Figure 31**). The jejunotomy is also performed using a monopolar device.

The running anterior barbed suture starts on the left side, incorporating the extramucosal layers of the jejunum and the full thickness of the esophageal wall (**Figure 32**).

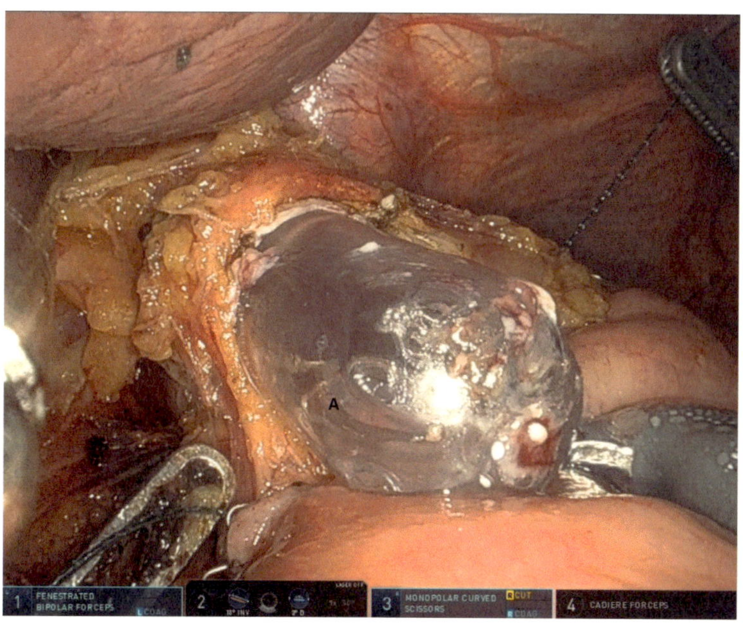

Figure 31.
Calibration of the gastrotomy during an NTG with a 42-Fr bougie (A).

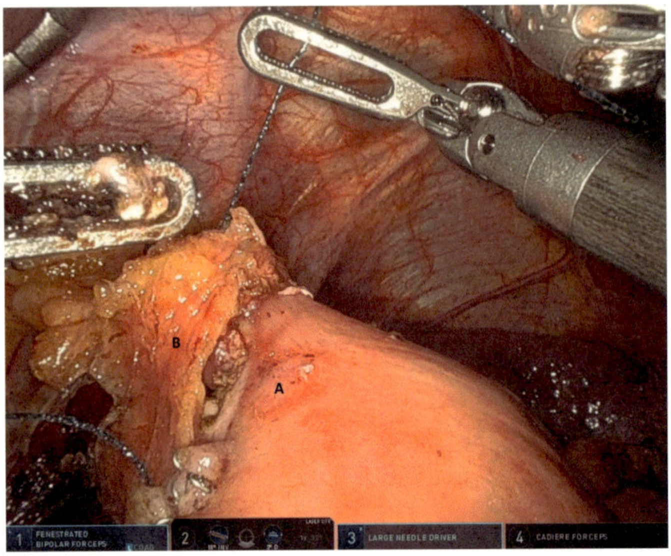

Figure 32.
Jejunum (A); gastric stump during NTG (B).

The anastomosis after NTG is technically the same realized between the small gastric pouch and the jejunum. The visualization of the Z line after the gastrotomy confirms that it is a very small gastric stump (**Figure 33**).

2.3.2 Petersen closing

The Petersen space is the mesenteric defect between the transverse mesocolon and the mesentery of the alimentary limb. This space is closed with a running 15-cm, 3/0 nonabsorbable barbed V-Loc® suture (Covidien, USA) right after the alimentary tract reconstruction (**Figure 34**).

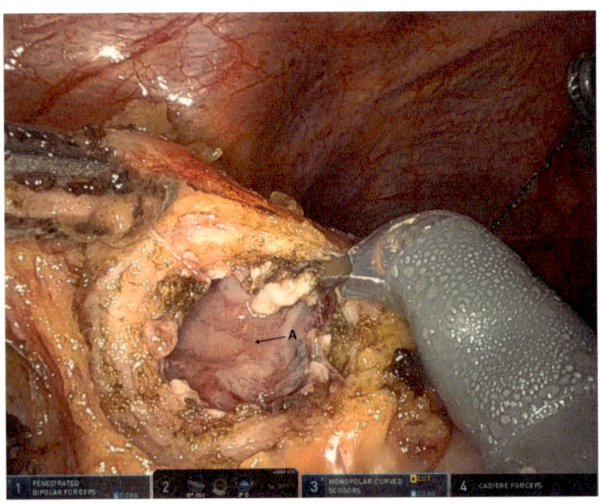

Figure 33.
Visualization of the Z line (A).

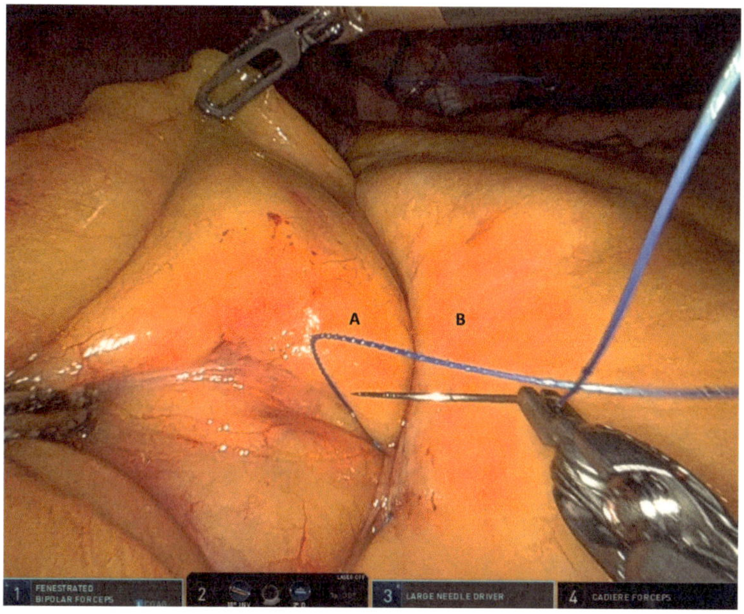

Figure 34.
Closing of the Petersen space between the transverse mesocolon (A) and the mesentery of the alimentary limb (B).

2.3.3 Jejuno-Jejunostomy

The omega loop is transformed into a Roux-en-Y after the transection of the jejunal loop 2 cm to the left of the esophagojejunostomy (gastrojejunostomy in case of NTG) (**Figure 35**).

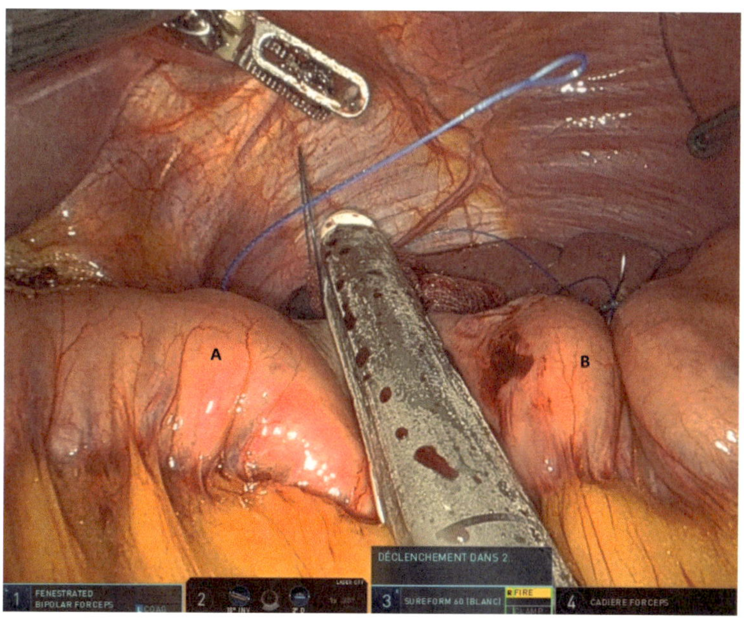

Figure 35.
Separation of the alimentary limb (A) and the bilio-pancreatic limb (B).

The jejunojejunostomy is then created using a 60-mm SureForm™ stapler (da Vinci Xi®, Intuitive) with a white cartridge. The enterotomy is closed with a 15-cm, 3/0 absorbable barbed V-Loc® suture (Covidien, USA) (**Figures 36–38**).

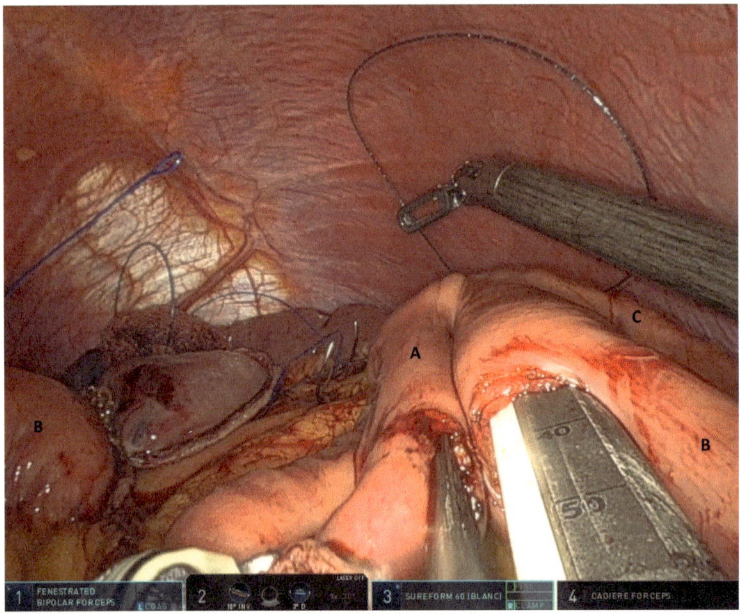

Figure 36.
Mechanical jejunojejunal anastomosis; bilio-pancreatic limb (A); alimentary limb (B); common limb (C).

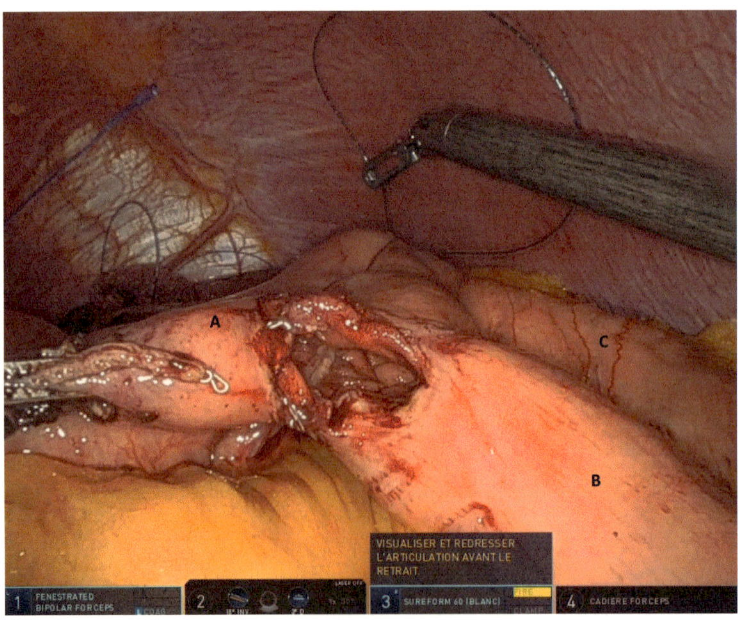

Figure 37.
Closing of the defect of jejunojejunostomy; bilio-pancreatic limb (A); alimentary limb (B); common limb (C).

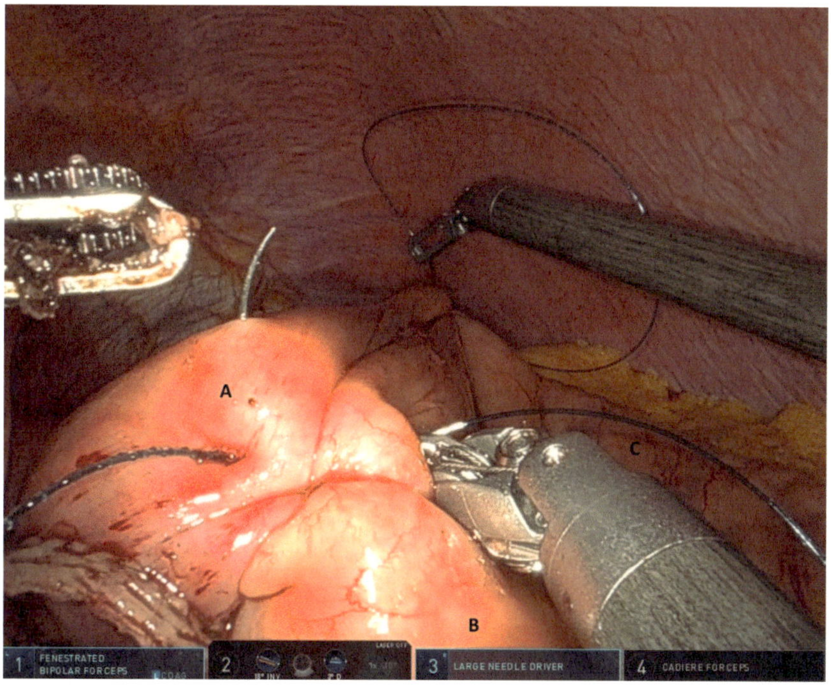

Figure 38.
Closing of the Jejunojenual anastomosis; bilio-pancreatic limb (A); alimentary limb (B); common limb (C).

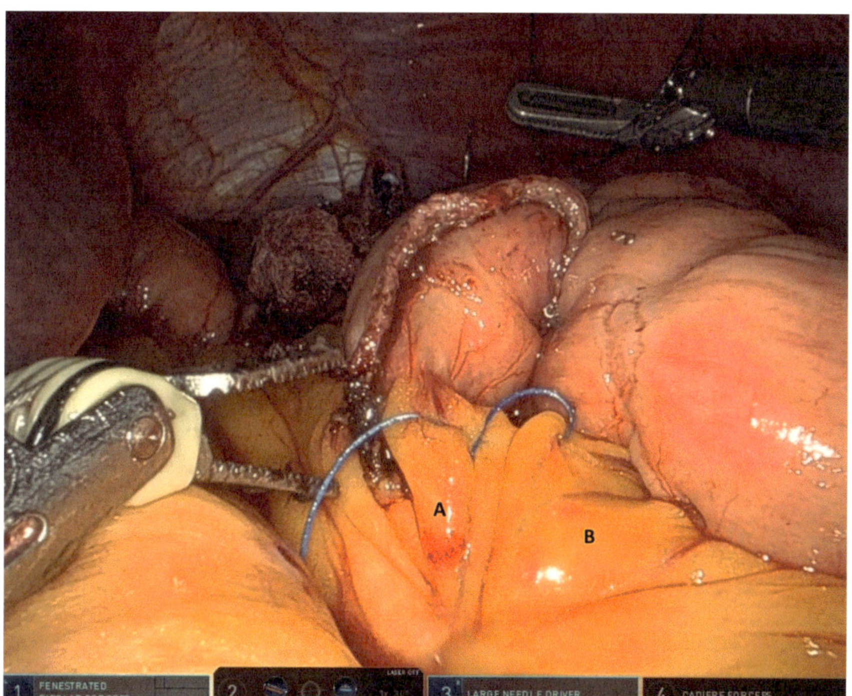

Figure 39.
Closing of the mesenteric defect between the mesentery of the bilio-pancreatic limb (A) and the mesentery of the alimentary limb (B).

2.3.4 Mesenteric defect closing

The last step of the operation consists of the closing of the mesenteric defect using a 15-cm, 3/0 nonabsorbable barbed V-Loc® suture (Covidien, USA) (**Figure 39**).

Specimen extraction is achieved through a Pfannenstiel incision.

No drain or nasogastric tube are left at the end of the procedure, and the patient starts oral intake on the first postoperative day.

Author details

Beniamino Pascotto*, Martine Goergen and Juan Santiago Azagra
General and Minimally Invasive (Laparoscopic and Robotic) Surgery Department, Centre Hospitalier de Luxembourg, Luxembourg

*Address all correspondence to: ben.pascotto@gmail.com

References

[1] Kitano S, Iso Y, Moriyama M, Sugimachi K. Laparoscopy-assisted Billroth I gastrectomy. Surgical Laparoscopy & Endoscopy. 1994;**4**(2):146-148

[2] Lee H-J, Hyung WJ, Yang H-K, Han SU, Park Y-K, An JY, et al. Short-term outcomes of a multicenter randomized controlled trial comparing laparoscopic distal gastrectomy with D2 lymphadenectomy to open distal gastrectomy for locally advanced gastric cancer (KLASS-02-RCT). Annals of Surgery. 2019;**270**(6):983-991

[3] Katai H, Mizusawa J, Katayama H, Takagi M, Yoshikawa T, Fukagawa T, et al. Short-term surgical outcomes from a phase III study of laparoscopy-assisted versus open distal gastrectomy with nodal dissection for clinical stage IA/IB gastric cancer: Japan clinical oncology group study JCOG0912. Gastric Cancer: Official Journal of the International Gastric Cancer Association: Japanese Gastric Cancer Association. 2017;**20**(4):699-708

[4] Shi Y, Xu X, Zhao Y, Qian F, Tang B, Hao Y, et al. Short-term surgical outcomes of a randomized controlled trial comparing laparoscopic versus open gastrectomy with D2 lymph node dissection for advanced gastric cancer. Surgical Endoscopy. 2018;**32**(5):2427-2433

[5] Yu J, Huang C, Sun Y, Su X, Cao H, Hu J, et al. Effect of laparoscopic vs open distal gastrectomy on 3-year disease-free survival in patients with locally advanced gastric cancer: The CLASS-01 randomized clinical trial. Journal of the American Medical Association. 2019;**321**(20):1983-1992

[6] Kim W, Kim H-H, Han S-U, Kim M-C, Hyung WJ, Ryu SW, et al. Decreased morbidity of laparoscopic distal gastrectomy compared with open distal gastrectomy for stage I gastric cancer: Short-term outcomes from a multicenter randomized controlled trial (KLASS-01). Annals of Surgery. 2016;**263**(1):28-35

[7] Azagra JS, Goergen M. Laparoscopic total gastrectomy. In: Meinero M, Melotti G, Mouret PH, editors. Laparoscopic Surgery – The Nineties. MASSON; 1994

[8] Ramos MFKP, Pereira MA, Dias AR, Ribeiro UJ, Zilberstein B, Nahas SC. Laparoscopic gastrectomy for early and advanced gastric cancer in a western center: A propensity score-matched analysis. Updates in Surgery. 2021;**73**(5):1867-1877

[9] Yuu K, Tsuchihashi K, Toyoda S, Kawasaki M, Kameyama M. Laparoscopic *vs.* open distal gastrectomy for advanced gastric cancer in elderly patients: A retrospective study. Mini-invasive Surgery. 2019;**3**(6). DOI: 10.20517/2574-1225.2018.73

[10] Azagra JS, Goergen M, Arru L, Facy O. Total gastrectomy for locally advanced cancer: The pure laparoscopic approach. Gastroenterology Report. 2013;**1**(2):119-126

[11] Azagra JS, Sarriugarte A, Ibañez FJ. Current status of gastrectomy for cancer: "Less is often more". Cirugia Espanola. Spain. 2018;**96**:603-605

[12] Kelly KJ, Selby L, Chou JF, Dukleska K, Capanu M, Coit DG, et al. Laparoscopic versus open gastrectomy for gastric adenocarcinoma in the west:

A case-control study. Annals of Surgical Oncology. 2015;**22**(11):3590-3596

[13] Popiela T, Kulig J, Kolodziejczyk P, Sierzega M. Long-term results of surgery for early gastric cancer. The British Journal of Surgery. 2002;**89**(8):1035-1042

[14] Chevallay M, Jung M, Berlth F, Seung-Hun C, Morel P, Mönig S. Laparoscopic surgery for gastric cancer: The European point of view. Journal of Oncology. 2019;**2019**:8738502

[15] Zhu Z, Li L, Xu J, Ye W, Zeng J, Chen B, et al. Laparoscopic versus open approach in gastrectomy for advanced gastric cancer: A systematic review. World Journal of Surgical Oncology. 2020;**18**(1):126

[16] Wei Y, Yu D, Li Y, Fan C, Li G. Laparoscopic versus open gastrectomy for advanced gastric cancer: A meta-analysis based on high-quality retrospective studies and clinical randomized trials. Clinics and Research in Hepatology and Gastroenterology. 2018;**42**(6):577-590

[17] Azagra JS, Goergen M, De Simone P, Ibañez-Aguirre J. Minimally invasive surgery for gastric cancer. Surgical Endoscopy. 1999;**13**(4):351-357

[18] Umemura A, Koeda K, Sasaki A, Fujiwara H, Kimura Y, Iwaya T, et al. Totally laparoscopic total gastrectomy for gastric cancer: Literature review and comparison of the procedure of esophagojejunostomy. Asian Journal of Surgery. 2015;**38**(2):102-112

[19] Lee S, Lee H, Song JH, Choi S, Cho M, Son T, et al. Intracorporeal esophagojejunostomy using a linear stapler in laparoscopic total gastrectomy: Comparison with circular stapling technique. BMC Surgery. 2020;**20**(1):100

[20] Huang C, Zhao J, Liu Z, Huang J, Zhu Z. Esophageal suspension method for hand-sewn esophagojejunostomy after totally laparoscopic total gastrectomy: A simple, safe, and feasible suturing technique. Frontiers in Oncology. 2020;**10**:575

[21] Norero E, Muñoz R, Ceroni M, Manzor M, Crovari F, Gabrielli M. Two-layer hand-sewn esophagojejunostomy in totally laparoscopic total gastrectomy for gastric cancer. Journal of Gastric Cancer. 2017;**17**(3):267-276

[22] Chen K, Wu D, Pan Y, Cai J-Q, Yan J-F, Chen D-W, et al. Totally laparoscopic gastrectomy using intracorporeally stapler or hand-sewn anastomosis for gastric cancer: A single-center experience of 478 consecutive cases and outcomes. World Journal of Surgical Oncology. 2016;**14**:115

[23] So KO, Park J-M. Totally laparoscopic total gastrectomy using intracorporeally hand-sewn esophagojejunostomy. Journal of Gastric Cancer. 2011;**11**(4):206-211

[24] Japanese gastric cancer treatment guidelines 2018 (5th edition). Gastric Cancer: Official Journal of the International Gastric Cancer Association: Japanese Gastric Cancer Association. 2021;**24**(1):1-21

[25] De Manzoni G, Marrelli D, Baiocchi GL, Morgagni P, Saragoni L, Degiuli M, et al. The Italian Research Group for Gastric Cancer (GIRCG) guidelines for gastric cancer staging and treatment: 2015. Gastric Cancer: Official Journal of the International Gastric Cancer Association: Japanese Gastric Cancer Association. 2017;**20**(1):20-30

[26] Jeong O, Park YK. Intracorporeal circular stapling esophagojejunostomy using the transorally inserted anvil

(OrVil) after laparoscopic total gastrectomy. Surgical Endoscopy. 2009;**23**(11):2624-2630

[27] Kim H-I, Cho I, Jang D-S, Hyung WJ. Intracorporeal esophagojejunostomy using a circular stapler with a new purse-string suture technique during laparoscopic total gastrectomy. Journal of the American College of Surgeons. 2013;**216**(2):e11-e16

[28] Kwon IG, Son Y-G, Ryu SW. Novel intracorporeal esophagojejunostomy using linear staplers during laparoscopic total gastrectomy: Π-shaped esophagojejunostomy, 3-in-1 technique. Journal of the American College of Surgeons. 2016;**223**(3):e25-e29

[29] Du J, Xue H, Zhao L, Hua J, Hu J, Zhang Z. Intracorporeal circular-stapled anastomosis after totally laparoscopic gastrectomy: A novel, simplest u-shaped parallel purse-string suture technique. Journal of Surgical Oncology. 2019;**120**(3):501-507

[30] Dulucq J-L, Wintringer P, Perissat J, Mahajna A. Completely laparoscopic total and partial gastrectomy for benign and malignant diseases: A single institute's prospective analysis. Journal of the American College of Surgeons. 2005;**200**(2):191-197

[31] Usui S, Nagai K, Hiranuma S, Takiguchi N, Matsumoto A, Sanada K. Laparoscopy-assisted esophagoenteral anastomosis using endoscopic purse-string suture instrument "Endo-PSI (II)" and circular stapler. Gastric Cancer: Official Journal of the International Gastric Cancer Association: Japanese Gastric Cancer Association. 2008;**11**(4):233-237

[32] Takagi H, Morimoto T. Near-total gastrectomy. Journal of Surgical Oncology. 1984;**26**(1):14-16

[33] Saario I, Salo J, Lempinen M, Kivilaakso E. Total and near-total gastrectomy for gastric cancer in patients over 70 years of age. American Journal of Surgery. 1987;**154**(3):269-270

[34] Salo JA, Saario I, Kivilaakso EOLM. Near-total gastrectomy for gastric cancer. American Journal of Surgery. 1988;**155**(3):486-489

[35] Arru L, Azagra JS, Facy O, Makkai-Popa ST, Poulain V, Goergen M. Totally laparoscopic 95% gastrectomy for cancer: Technical considerations. Langenbeck's Archives Surgery. 2015;**400**(3):387-393

[36] Sarriugarte A, Arru L, Makai-Popa S, Goergen M, Ibañez-Aguirre FJ, Azagra JS. Short-term results of near-total (95%) laparoscopic gastrectomy. Cirugía Española. 2018;**96**(10):634-639

[37] Facy O, Arru L, Azagra JS. Intestinal anastomosis after laparoscopic total gastrectomy. Journal of Visceral Surgery. 2012;**149**(3):e179-e184

[38] Azagra JS, Pascotto B, Arru L, Ibañez FJ, Makkai-Popa ST, Goergen M. Hand-sewn anastomosis after 95{\%} gastrectomy, total gastrectomy, and total gastrectomy extended to the distal esophagus for gastric cancer. In: Asunción Acosta M, Cuesta MA, Bruna M, editors. Atlas of Minimally Invasive Techniques in Upper Gastrointestinal Surgery. Cham: Springer International Publishing; 2021. pp. 323-332. DOI: 10.1007/978-3-030-55176-6_40

[39] Pascotto B, González González L, Di Saverio S, Arru L, Goergen M, Azagra JS. Minimally invasive hand-sewn barbed anastomosis after total and near-total gastrectomy: standardized Azagra's technique. Journal of Gastrointestinal Surgery: Official Journal of the Society for Surgery of the Alimentary Tract. 2023;**27**(5):990-991

[40] Salvador-Rosés H, Escartín A, Muriel P, Santamaría M, González M, Jara J, et al. Robotic versus open approach in total gastrectomy for gastric cancer: A comparative single-center study of perioperative outcomes. Journal of Robotic Surgery. 2023;**17**(4):1735-1741

[41] Trastulli S, Desiderio J, Lin J-X, Reim D, Zheng C-H, Borghi F, et al. Open vs robotic gastrectomy with D2 lymphadenectomy: A propensity score-matched analysis on 1469 patients from the IMIGASTRIC prospective database. Langenbeck's Archives Surgery. 2023;**408**(1):302

[42] Marano L, Cwalinski T, Girnyi S, Skokowski J, Goyal A, Malerba S, et al. Evaluating the role of robotic surgery gastric cancer treatment: A comprehensive review by the robotic global surgical society (TROGSS) and European Federation International Society for Digestive Surgery (EFISDS) joint working group. Current Oncology. 2025;**32**(2)